Lynda Aoudia

Benign breast tumors

Lynda Aoudia

Benign breast tumors

Imprint
Any brand names and product names mentioned in this book are subject to trademark, brand or patent protection and are trademarks or registered trademarks of their respective holders. The use of brand names, product names, common names, trade names, product descriptions etc. even without a particular marking in this work is in no way to be construed to mean that such names may be regarded as unrestricted in respect of trademark and brand protection legislation and could thus be used by anyone.

Cover image: www.ingimage.com

This book is a translation from the original published under ISBN 978-620-6-71295-4.

Publisher:
Sciencia Scripts
is a trademark of
Dodo Books Indian Ocean Ltd. and OmniScriptum S.R.L publishing group

120 High Road, East Finchley, London, N2 9ED, United Kingdom
Str. Armeneasca 28/1, office 1, Chisinau MD-2012, Republic of Moldova, Europe
Printed at: see last page
ISBN: 978-620-7-94586-3

Benign breast tumors

Lynda AOUDIA

Foreword

Benign breast tumors comprise a heterogeneous group of lesions, symptoms and imaging aspects. The majority of breast lesions are benign. The aim of diagnosing these tumors is always to rule out a malignant lesion, or at least one at risk of degeneration.
A good understanding of these tumors helps to ensure appropriate management.

This book is designed primarily for radiologists involved in breast imaging.

Prof. Lynda AOUDIA

Table of contents

Introduction 4

Anatomical reminder 5

1. Breast anatomy 5

2. Galactophoric tree 5

Histological reminder 7

Benign tumors 8

1. Fibroadenomas 8

2. Phyllodes tumors 36

3. Papilloma 49

4. Adenomyepithelioma 53

5. Pseudoangiomatous stromal hyperplasia *(PASH)* 55

6. Hamartome 60

7. Rarer benign tumours 65

References 69

Introduction

Benign breast tumors are important to know about for several reasons:

- They are very common and can give rise to a wide range of clinical symptoms, requiring investigations to confirm their benign nature and sometimes justify specific treatment modalities;

- they are more often discovered by chance in the context of breast cancer screening; it is therefore important to be able to gather arguments in favour of benignity to reduce patient anxiety, but also to avoid further explorations, follow-up and unnecessary surgery;

- Atypical or misleading aspects may pose problems of differential diagnosis with malignant pathology.

Benign breast tumors are dominated by fibroadenomas. **Other, rarer tumors may pose problems of etiological diagnosis.**

In the majority of cases, mammography and ultrasound can be used to diagnose these tumors. MRI can be a useful adjunct in certain cases where diagnosis is problematic. Guided sampling techniques are used to rule out malignant lesions.

Anatomical reminder

1. Breast anatomy

The breast is a globular organ occupying the anterior-superior part of the thorax. It lies on top of the pectoralis muscle, which provides support [1]. It consists mainly of a mammary gland, supportive connective tissue and adipose tissue, all covered by the skin. The apex of the breast is represented by the nipple surrounded by the areola (fig. 1). It is made up of some fifteen main galactophores, each delimiting a lobe. The milk ducts open into the nipple at the level of the milk pores, after dilating slightly to form a lactiferous sinus.

Thin fibrous partitions separate the lobes, extending from the anterior surface of the gland into the dermis to form Cooper's ligaments and Duret's ridges (fig. 1).

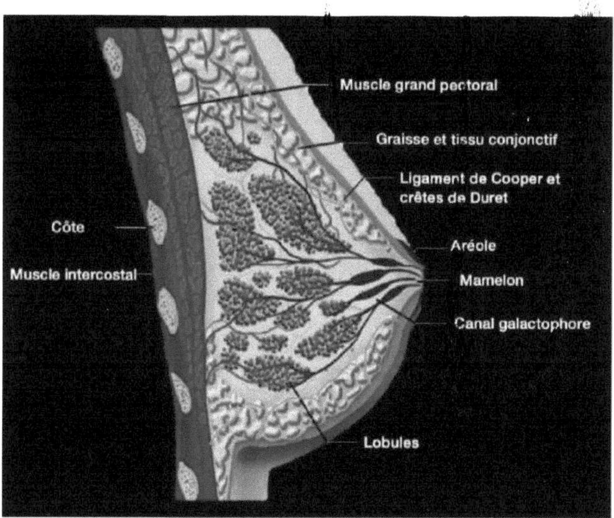

Fig. 1. anatomical structure of the breast.

2. Galactophoric tree

The breast is made up of some fifteen main milk ducts, which end in a nipple pore.

These main ducts, after a dilatation known as the lactiferous sinus, branch out into secondary ducts of medium and small caliber up to the Ductulo-Lobular Terminal Unit (DLTU).

This UDTL consists of an extra- and intra-lobular terminal galactophore and a lobule made up of ten or so alveoli called acini. The UDTL is embedded in a loose connective tissue known as pallaeal tissue. All this tissue is surrounded by adipose tissue (fig. 2).

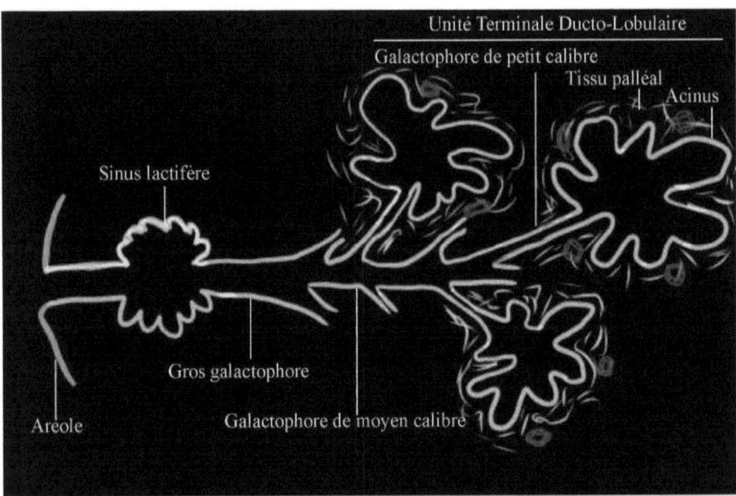

Fig. 2: Diagram of the galactophoric tree.

Histological reminder

The entire galactophoric tree is made up of a double cell bed resting on a basement membrane in direct contact with the blood vessels (fig. 3):

- an inner layer of columnar epithelial cells, responsible for the milk secretory function.
- an outer layer of myoepithelial cells responsible for contraction.

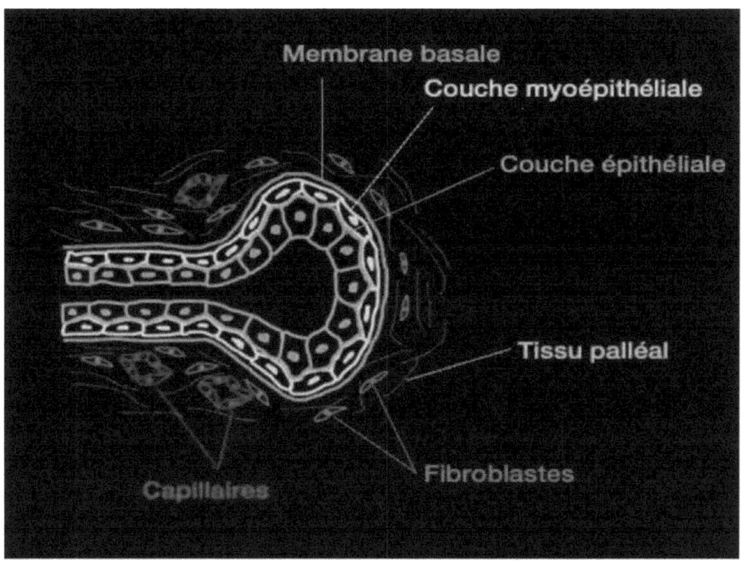

Fig. 3: Histological diagram of acinar constituents.

Benign tumors

1. Fibroadenomas

Fibroadenomas are the most common benign breast lesions in young women [2]. A hormone-dependent tumour, it increases in volume during pregnancy and breastfeeding, and decreases during the perimenopausal period [3]. Use of oral contraceptives before the age of 20 increases the risk of developing fibroadenomas [4]. Usually discovered incidentally during ultrasound examination.

Most fibroadenomas have similar imaging findings and these lesions can be defined as simple fibroadenomas. However, due to different histopathological features and components, histological variants of fibroadenomas have been described. These variants include juvenile, giant, complex, myxoid and hyalinized fibroadenomas. These different fibroadenoma subtypes have distinct clinical manifestations, malignant transformation potential and therapeutic strategies.

1.1. Epidemiology

Fibroadenomas tend to appear at an early age. It is most often seen in adolescent girls, and less often in post-menopausal women. The incidence of fibroadenoma decreases with age, generally occurring before the age of 30 in women in the general population, with a peak incidence between the ages of 20 and 24 estimated at 115/100,000 woman-years [5]. It is estimated that 10% of the world's female population will suffer from a fibroadenoma at least once in their lives.

1.2. Pathogenesis

Fibroadenoma is a cellular proliferation of the connective and epithelial tissue of the terminal canal-lobular unit [6, 7].

In some cases, fibroadenomas may express estrogen and progesterone receptors.

Estrogen and progesterone stimulate hormone receptors in fibroadenomas, leading to excessive proliferation of connective and epithelial cells. During the menopause, fibroadenomas undergo atrophy as circulating levels of these female hormones fall.

Epidermal growth factor (EGF) receptors may be expressed in some fibroadenomas [8].

The mediator complex subunit 12 (MED12) gene is involved in fibroadenoma genesis. The MED12 gene contributes to the production of the MED12 protein, which, along with other proteins, is essential for eukaryotic transcriptional regulation [9, 10].

In over 70% of cases, fibroadenomas present as a single mass, and multiple masses in 10% to 25% [11].

Most fibroadenomas develop in the upper external quadrants. The size of fibroadenomas can vary with the menstrual cycle and circulating hormone levels.

1.3. Clinic

The fibroadenoma most often presents as a well-limited, regularly contoured, round or oval, firm mass, mobile in relation to the deep plane, painless, varying in size from a few millimetres to a few centimetres [12]. The time course of fibroadenomas is unpredictable. Generally, they appear in adolescence, with a possible increase in size, up to 2 to 3 cm in one year, followed by a decrease in 40% of cases, stability in 30% of fibroadenomas and progression in 30% of cases [13].

1.4. Histology

1.4.1. Macroscopy

Oval or lobulated, circumscribed mass with variable consistency depending on composition: elastic in young girls, firmer or even hard in older women (hyaline involution, calcification) (fig. 4) [14].

The cross-sectional edge of the mass is beige in color, with a solid consistency and slit-shaped spaces (fig. 4).

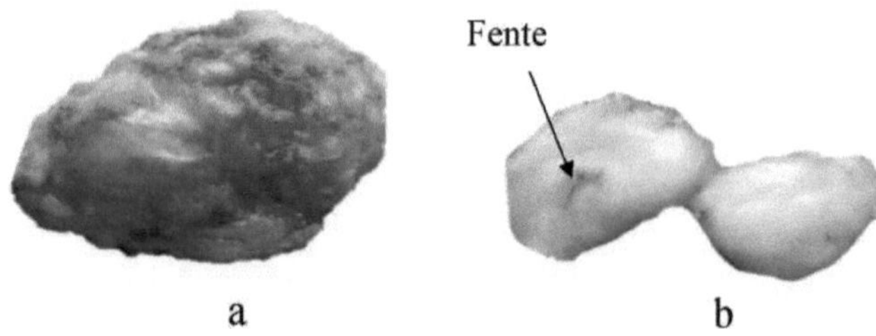

Fig. 4: Fibroadenoma (a) Macroscopy. (b) Cross-sectional slice. Circumscribed, oval mass with lobulated contours.

1.4.2. Microscopy

A tumor with a dual connective (mesenchymal) and epithelial component. The conjunctival component is fibrous, often sparsely cellular, sometimes myxoid. The epithelial component contains glandular cavities with often stretched, sometimes virtual lumens, lined by a double cellular base, epithelial and myoepithelial (fig. 5).

There are two varieties:

- In pericanal fibroadenoma, the proliferation of ducts retains a circular lumen, and there is also connective tissue hyperplasia (fig. 6).

- Intracanal fibroadenoma the tumor presents stretched, collapsed ducts with arciform contours, secondary to conjunctival hyperplasia that pushes back the ducts (fig. 6).

Peripherally, the fibroadenoma has regular, symmetrical boundaries, with a conjunctival pseudocapsule surrounding the lesion and separating it from normal breast tissue, giving the so-called "pushing" appearance (fig. 7).

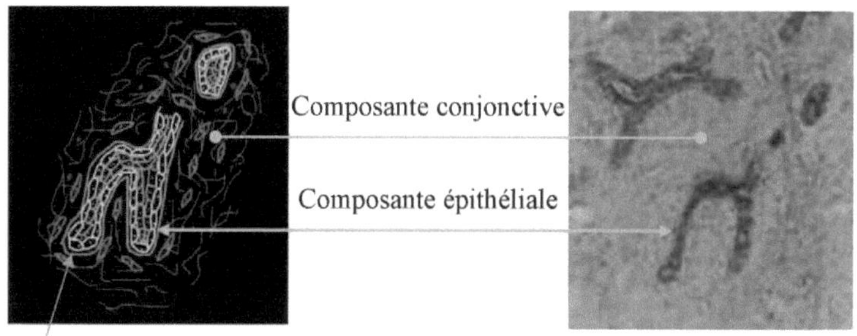

Fig. 5. Fibroadenoma. Microscopy.

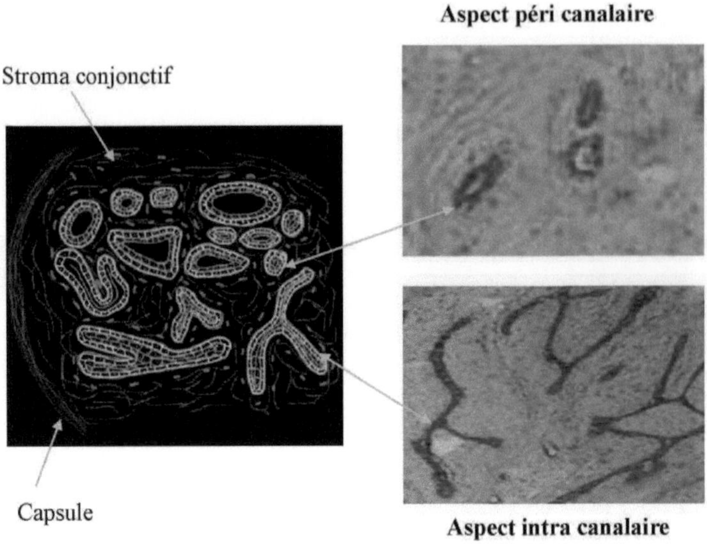

Fig. 6. fibroadenoma. Microscopy. Peri- and intracanal aspect.

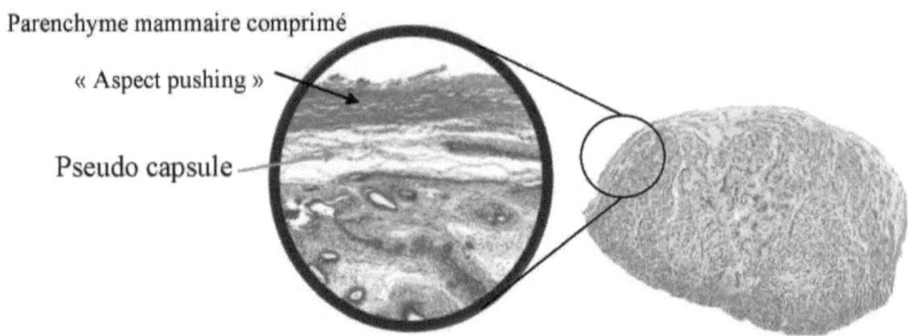

Fig. 7. Fibroadenoma. Microscopy. The conjunctival pseudocapsule surrounding the lesion and separating it from normal breast tissue, with a "pushing" appearance [15].

1.3. Imaging

1.5.1. Simple fibroadenoma

The simple fibroadenoma is classified in the ANDI classification as a simple "aberration" from normal. This benign tumor is most common in girls under 25, and generally appears in the first few years after menarche. There is a peak at age 20, with incidence peaking between the ages of 20 and 30. Fibroadenoma appears to be more common in the Indian and African populations [16].

The simple fibroadenoma most often presents as a well-limited mass measuring around 1 to 3 cm.

On histology, tumor proliferation shows no stromal cellular atypia or mitosis, and stromal cellularity is similar to that of perilobular stroma [17] (fig. 8).

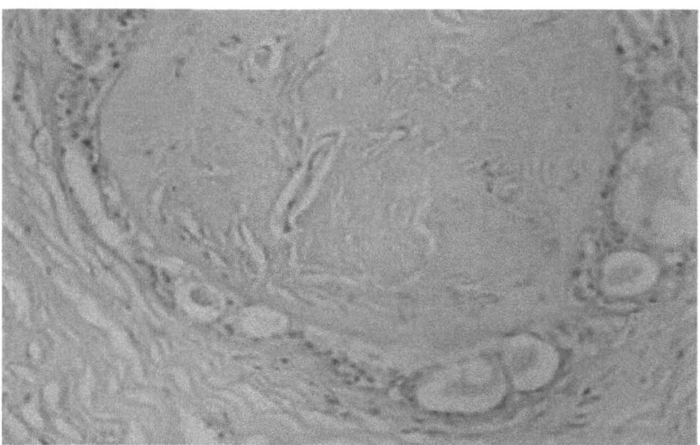

Fig. 8. simple fibroadenoma. Histology. Tumor proliferation shows no stromal cellular atypia or mitosis.

1.5.1.1. Mammography

Mammography can be nonsensitive and non-specific in young women, due to breast density.

On mammography, a simple fibroadenoma appears as a mass, round or oval, with circumscribed or macrolobulated contours, isodense or hyperdense. A clear perilesional halo sign is frequently observed due to the Mach effect, which corresponds to the peripheral arrangement of connective tissue that, under tension, forms a fibrous lamina or pseudocapsule (fig. 9).

Nevertheless, mammography findings often overlap with the imaging of other benign lesions, such as cysts. As a result, an additional imaging method, usually ultrasound, is performed.

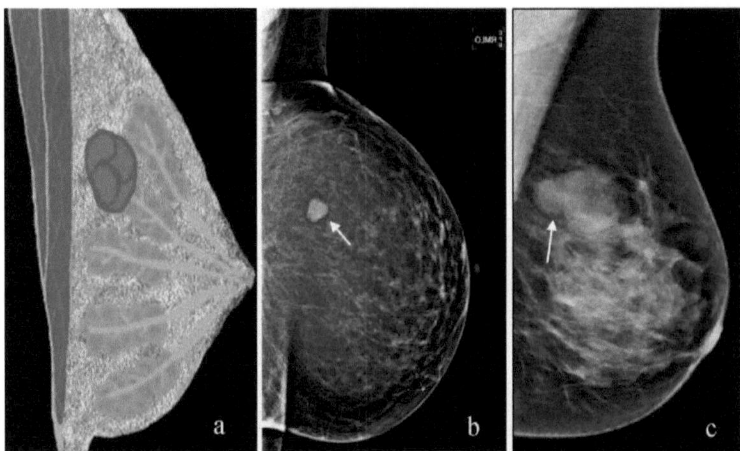

Fig. 9. simple fibroadenoma. (a) Schematic diagram. (b+c) Mammogram. Round or oval mass, with circumscribed or macrolobulated contours, hyperdense or isodense with a clear perilesional "mach effect" halo (arrows).

1.5.1.2. B-mode ultrasound

Ultrasonography shows the characteristics of a fibroadenoma, in the form of an oval, homogeneous mass with circumscribed or macrolobulated contours, hypoechoic or isoechoic. An important feature of simple fibroadenomas on ultrasound is the skin-parallel orientation of the lesion, the normal anatomical orientation of the lobules (fig. 10). Another important sign of simple fibroadenoma is the echogenic fibrous internal septa [18] (fig.10). Due to compression of the mammary parenchyma by the lesion, an echogenic lateral pseudocapsule may form [19] (fig.10).

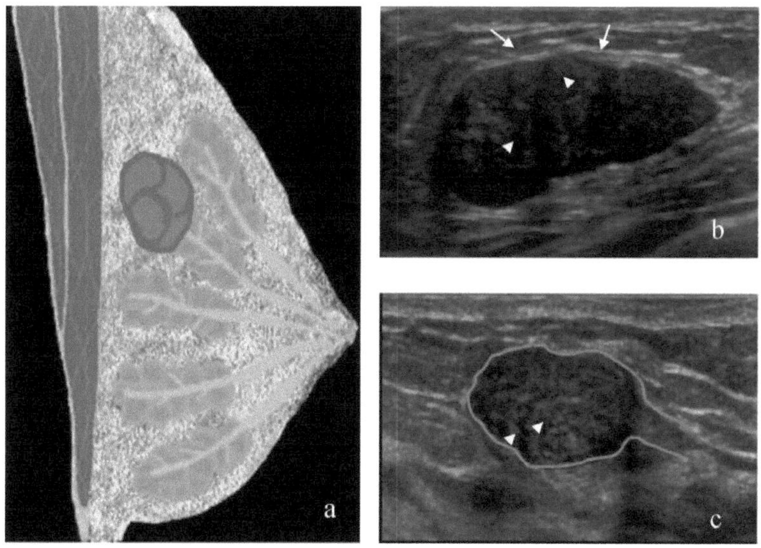

Fig. 10. simple fibroadenoma. (a) Schematic diagram. (b+c) Ultrasound. Oval, homogeneous mass with macrolobulated contours, hypoechoic, orientation parallel to the skin, showing echogenic internal septa (arrowheads), with a peripheral echogenic pseudocapsule (arrows).

1.5.1.3. Color Doppler

The majority of fibroadenomas show vascularization on color Doppler, in 80% of cases simple fibroadenomas [19, 20].

Three types of vessel have been described (fig. 11):

o Feeder vessels, which are prominent vessels that lead from the surrounding breast tissue to the fibroadenoma.

o Capsular vessels are located in the capsule.

o Segmental vessels are located in the fibrous septa of the fibroadenoma.

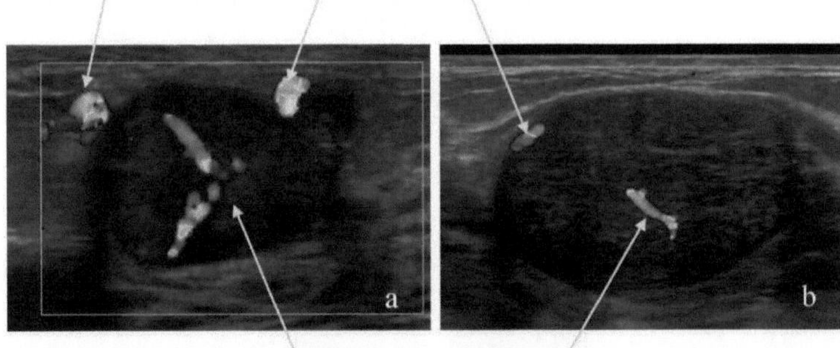

Fig. 11. Simple fibroadenoma. (a+b) Color Doppler. Vascularization.

1.5.1.4. Elastography

Simple fibroadenomas are generally soft on elastography, with elasticity scores ranging from 1 to 3 and low elasticity ratios (fig.12).

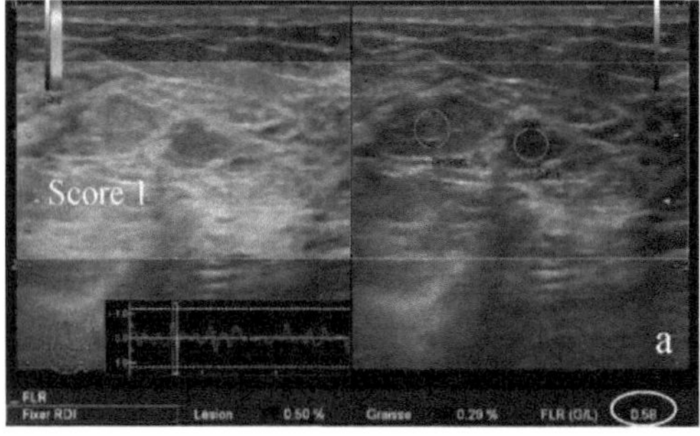

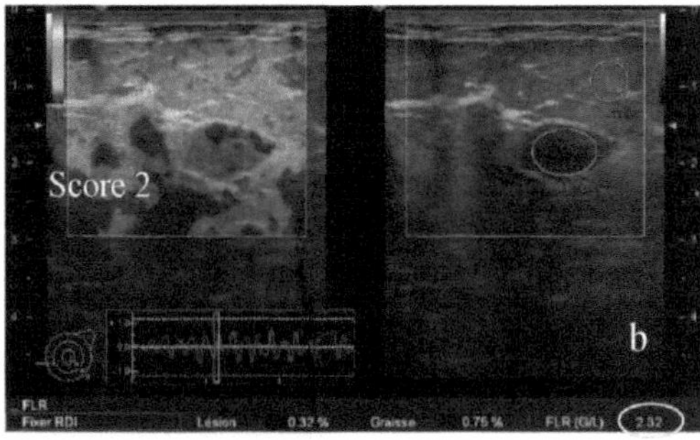

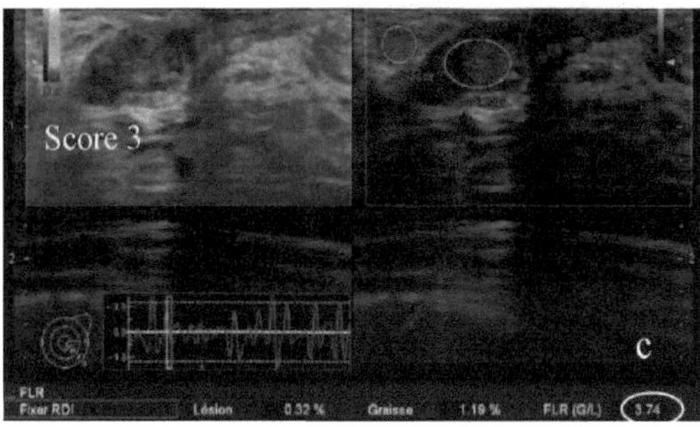

Fig. 12. Simple fibroadenoma. Elastography. (a) fibroadenoma scored 1 with an estimated low elasticity ratio of 0.58. (b) Scored fibroadenoma 2 with an estimated elasticity ratio of 2.32. (c) Scored fibroadenoma 3 with an elasticity ratio lower than that of a malignant lesion, estimated at 3.74.

1.5.1.5.MRI

Magnetic resonance imaging (MRI) findings of simple fibroadenomas also vary.

The shape and contours are similar to those seen on mammography and ultrasound.

On T1-weighted sequences, the lesion is isointense with the surrounding breast parenchyma. The signal on T2-weighted sequences changes according to the content of the lesion. In dynamic sequences, enhancement is generally progressive.

The most important MRI feature suggestive of fibroadenoma is the internal septa, hyposignal T1, T2, unenhanced after contrast injection in over 95% of cases. However, the absence of internal septa does not exclude the diagnosis of fibroadenoma [21] (fig. 13).

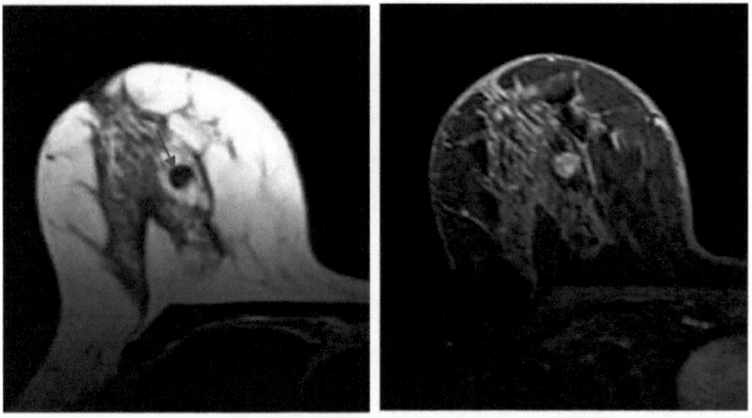

Fig. 13. Simple fibroadenoma. MRI: (a) T2 sequence; (b) T1 sequence with native injection. Round mass with circumscribed contours, in T2 hyposignal, showing septa in T2 hyposignal, not enhanced after injection of contrast medium (arrows).

1.5.2. Juvenile fibroadenoma

Juvenile fibroadenoma is a rare variant of fibroadenoma, accounting for 7-8% [2,

22]. Juvenile fibroadenomas are commonly seen in adolescents between the ages of 10 and 18, with African-American lesions often multiple and bilateral in this population [22, 23].

Macroscopically, the mass is generally circumscribed, often exceeding 3 cm [24]. Microscopic histopathology is characterized by a conjunctival component with increased cellularity, a fasciculated appearance and exceptional mitoses (<1/mm2). The epithelial component frequently shows ductal hyperplasia [25] (fig. 14).

Clinically, juvenile fibroadenomas appear as a painless mass that rapidly increases in size, causing breast hypertrophy or asymmetry [26, 27]. Superficial venous dilatation and skin ulceration may be observed [26] (fig. 15).

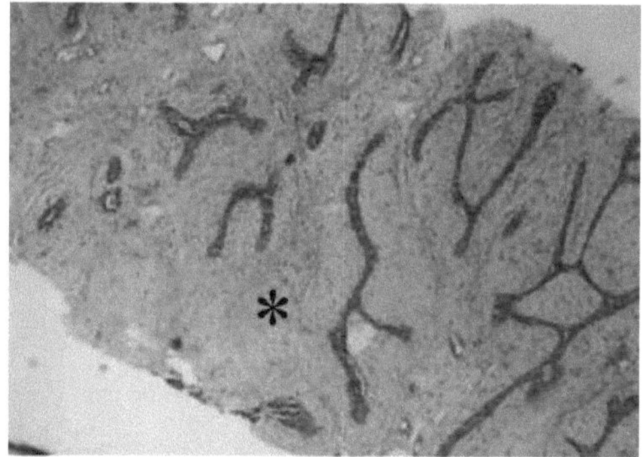

Fig. 14. Juvenile fibroadenoma. Histology. Hypercellular mesenchymal component (asterisk).

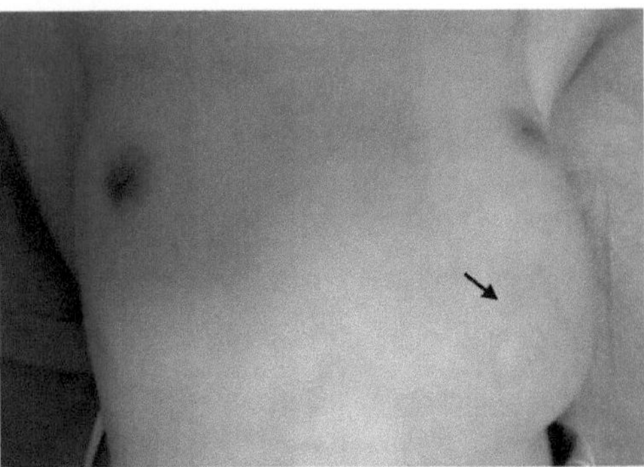

Fig. 15. Juvenile fibroadenoma. Left breast mass causing breast asymmetry. Superficial venous dilatation (arrow).

1.5.2.1.Imaging

As juvenile fibroadenomas are seen during adolescence, mammographic examination is neither recommended nor necessary [24].

Ultrasound is the main diagnostic test. The sonographic features of juvenile fibroadenomas are similar to those of simple fibroadenomas. The mass is oval, circumscribed, oriented parallel to the skin, with hypo- or isoechoic echotexture, often with posterior enhancement [28, 29] (fig. 16 a).

On color Doppler, fibroadenomas are hypervascularized [28] (fig. 16 b).

Elastography and MRI findings in juvenile fibroadenomas are similar to those in simple fibroadenomas (Fig. 16 c+d). On MRI, the masses are hyposignal on T1 sequences and hypersignal on T2-weighted sequences, reflecting the hypercellularity of the lesions, with hypointense internal septa that are not enhanced after contrast injection.

Patient age and lesion size >5 cm and clinical findings, are important features for the diagnosis of juvenile fibroadenomas [30].

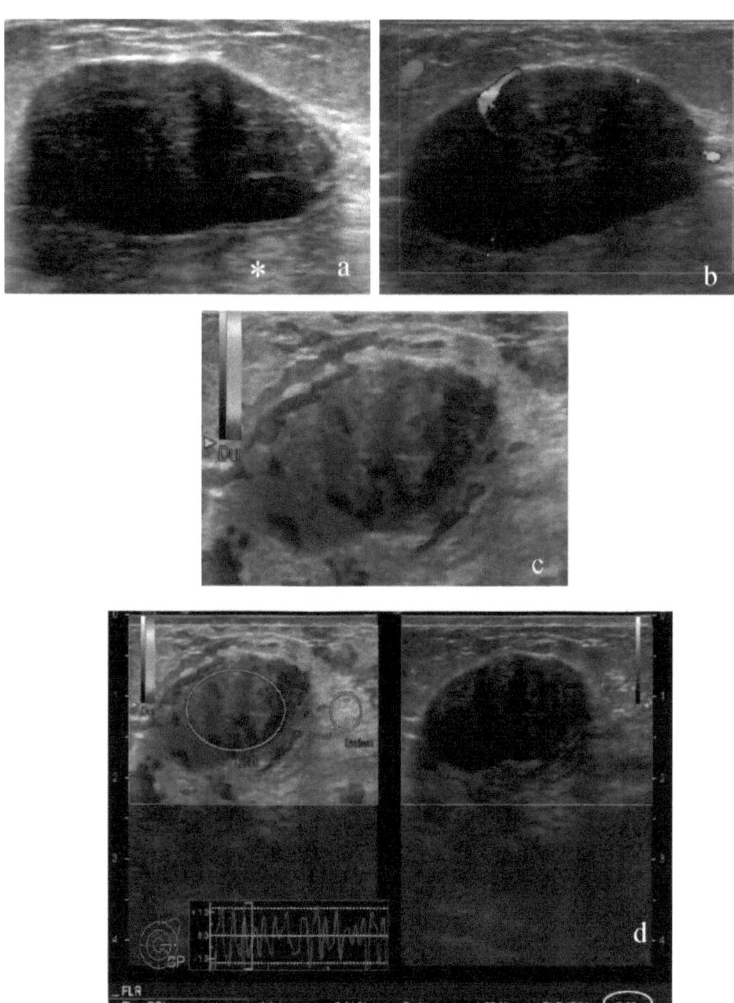

Fig. 16. Juvenile fibroadenoma. (a) B-mode ultrasound. Hypoechoic, circumscribed, homogeneous mass with horizontal long axis and peripheral pseudocapsule (arrow) and posterior enhancement (asterisk). (b) Colour Doppler. Peripheral vascularization is central. (c+d) Elastography. Soft mass, elasticity score 2 and elasticity ratio 2.29.

1.5.3. Giant fibroadenoma

Giant fibroadenoma is another rare variant, accounting for 0.5-2% of fibroadenomas [30]. Giant fibroadenomas are seen in pre-menopausal women [31]. In fact, juvenile fibroadenomas in patients aged 10-18 years eventually develop into giant fibroadenomas due to their rapid growth [32]. Giant fibroadenomas are large masses, over 5 cm, greater than 500g)[30, 33] Giant fibroadenomas are more common in African-American and East Asian women. Similar to juvenile fibroadenomas, rapid growth and can cause aesthetic problems of breast hypertrophy and asymmetry [27].

Imaging is similar to that of juvenile fibroadenoma (Fig. 17).

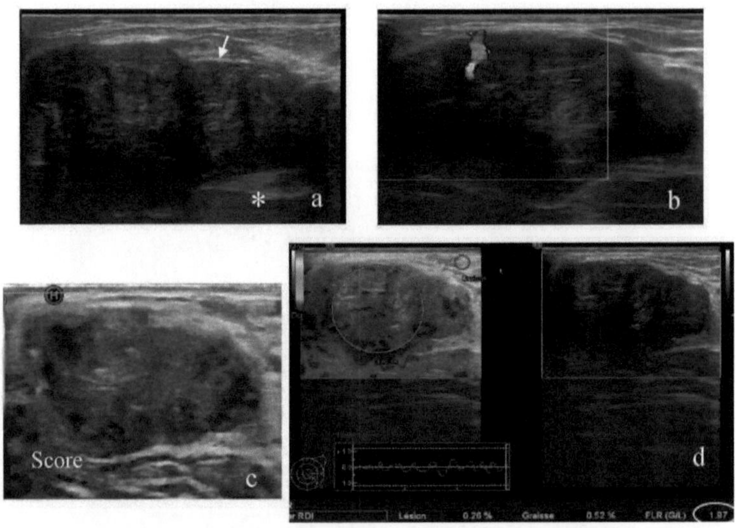

Fig. 17. Giant fibroadenoma. (a) B-mode ultrasound. Voluminous, hypoechoic, circumscribed, homogeneous mass with horizontal long axis, peripheral pseudocapsule (arrow) and posterior enhancement (asterisk). (b) Colour Doppler. Peripheral vascularization is central. (c+d) Elastography. Soft mass, elasticity score 2 and elasticity ratio 1.97.

1.5.3. Fibroadenoma complex

An important variant of the fibroadenoma is the complex fibroadenoma. First described by Dupont [34], fibroadenoma comprises at least one or more pathological features [35] :

> o Cysts > 3 mm.

> o Epithelial calcifications.

> o Sclerosing adenosis.

> o Apocrine metaplasia.

Complex fibroadenomas account for 22% of all fibroadenomas [35]. They increase the risk of infiltrating breast cancer by 3.1 times, and by 1.89 for simple fibroadenomas [36]. They require lumpectomy with safety margin. [37].

1.5.4.1.Imaging

On mammography, complex fibroadenomas usually appear as a circumscribed, round or oval mass. Coarse heterogeneous calcifications may be observed. In rare cases, focal asymmetry may be present [38].

On ultrasonography, the characteristics of complex fibroadenomas are similar to those on mammography [39]. Pinto et al. observed that most complex fibroadenomas are oval in shape, circumscribed, oriented parallel to the skin, without posterior acoustic effects or calcifications [40]. However, irregular shape, uncircumscribed contours, heterogeneous echostructure, presence of calcifications within it and posterior acoustic enhancement are more common in complex fibroadenomas than in other fibroadenoma variants [40]. These authors concluded that the most relevant features of complex fibroadenomas are an irregularly shaped mass, with microlobulated contours, orientation parallel to the skin, heterogeneous echostructure due to the presence of cysts < 3 mm and calcifications [40] (fig. 18).

To the best of our knowledge, there are no specific elastographic characteristics of complex fibroadenomas in the literature. The elasticity score for complex fibroadenomas is usually 1, 2 or 3 (fig. 19).

MRI findings in complex fibroadenomas are similar to those in simple fibroadenomas and other fibroadenoma variants, with no specific character.

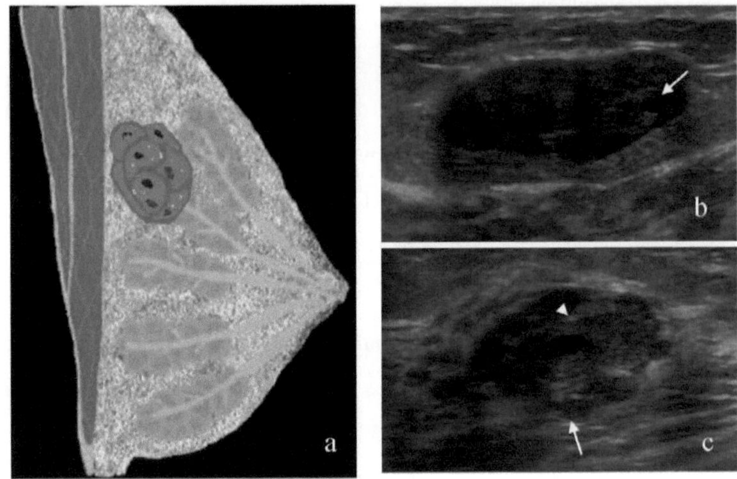

Fig. 18. Fibroadenoma complex (a) Schematic diagram. (b+c) B-mode ultrasonography. Hypoechoic mass, irregularly shaped, with microlobulated contours, heterogeneous echostructure by the presence of cysts < 3 mm (arrows) and calcifications (arrowhead).

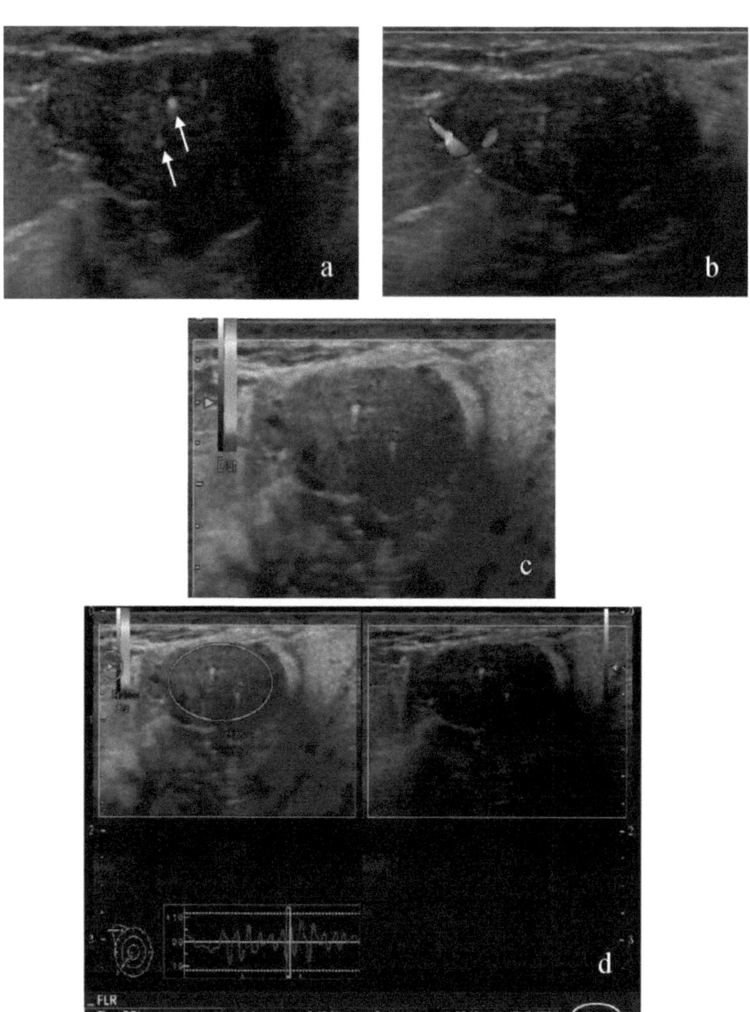

Fig. 19. **complex fibroadenoma** (a) B-mode ultrasonography: oval mass with microlobulated contours, long horizontal axis parallel to the skin, heterogeneous echostructure due to the presence of cysts (arrow) and

1.5.4. Myxoid fibroadenoma

Myxoid fibroadenoma is a histological subtype of fibroadenoma with abundant myxoid matrix and hypocellular stroma [41] (fig. 20). The myxoid fibroadenoma is often described in Carney syndrome [42], an autosomal dominant disease characterized by the association of pigmentary anomalies of the skin, myxomas (cardiac or cutaneous), tumors or dysfunctions of endocrine tumors and schwannomas [43, 44].

On imaging, mammographic and ultrasonographic findings are similar to those of simple fibroadenoma. Following a myxoid component of the stroma, a mass with significant posterior enhancement is often observed on ultrasound (fig. 21).

On MRI, myxoid fibroadenomas show a T1 hyopsignal and usually a T2 hypersignal. On dynamic sequences, rapid, homogeneous enhancement is often observed with a type 3 dynamic curve, responsible for false positives [45].

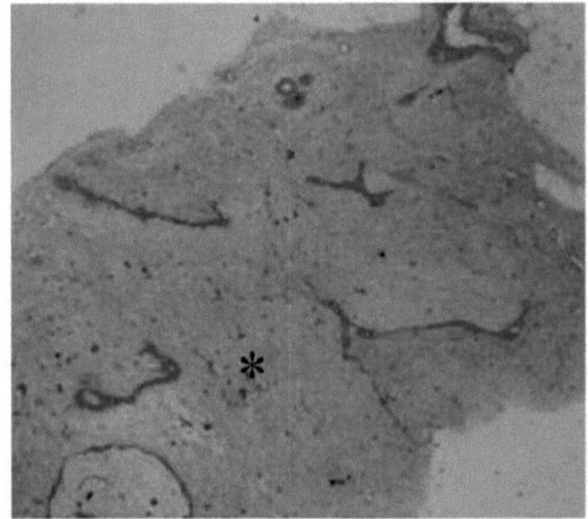

Fig. 20. Myxoid fibroadenoma. Histology. Mesenchymal component with hypocellular myxoid appearance (asterisk).

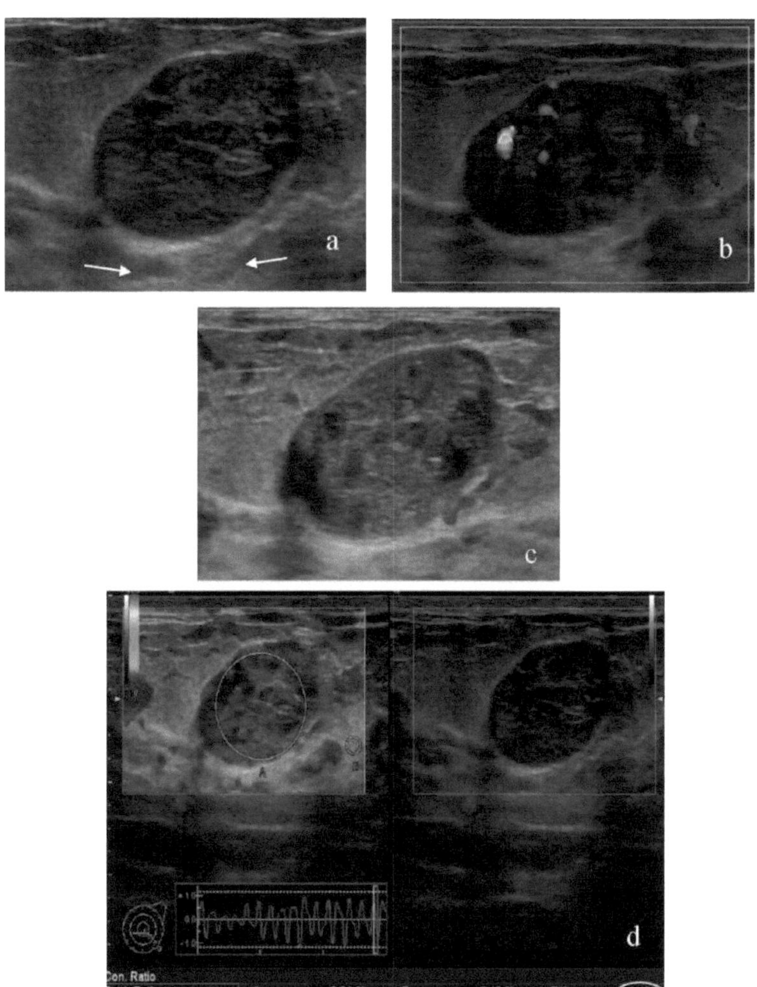

Fig. 21. myxoid fibroadenoma. (a) B-mode ultrasound. Oval mass with circumscribed contours, long horizontal axis parallel to the skin, homogeneous echostructure with posterior acoustic enhancement (arrows). (b) Colour Doppler. Peripheral vascularity is central. (c+d) Elastography. Soft mass, elasticity score 2 and low elasticity ratio of 1.43.

1.5.6. Cellular fibroadenoma

Cellular fibroadenoma is a variant of fibroadenoma characterized by high stromal cellularity that is uniform and without atypia [46, 47] (fig.22). Cellular fibroadenomas are generally observed in young women, and cellularity decreases with age [48]. Histologically, cellular fibroadenomas pose a diagnostic problem with low-grade phyllodes tumours [46]. There are no distinctive imaging features of cellular fibroadenomas (fig. 23).

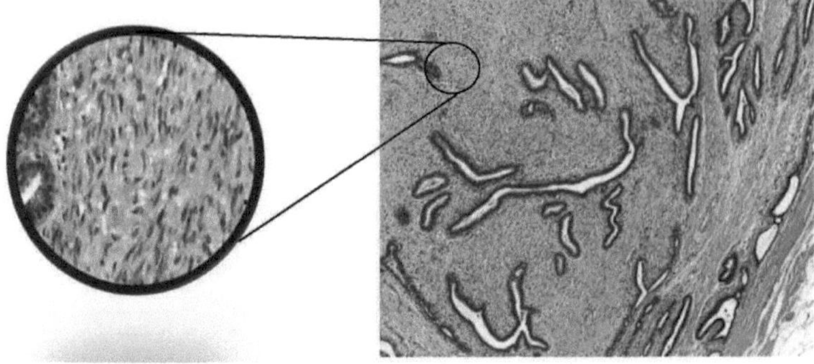

Fig. 22. Cellular fibroadenoma. Histology. Stromal hypercellularity. Uniform, without atypia [48].

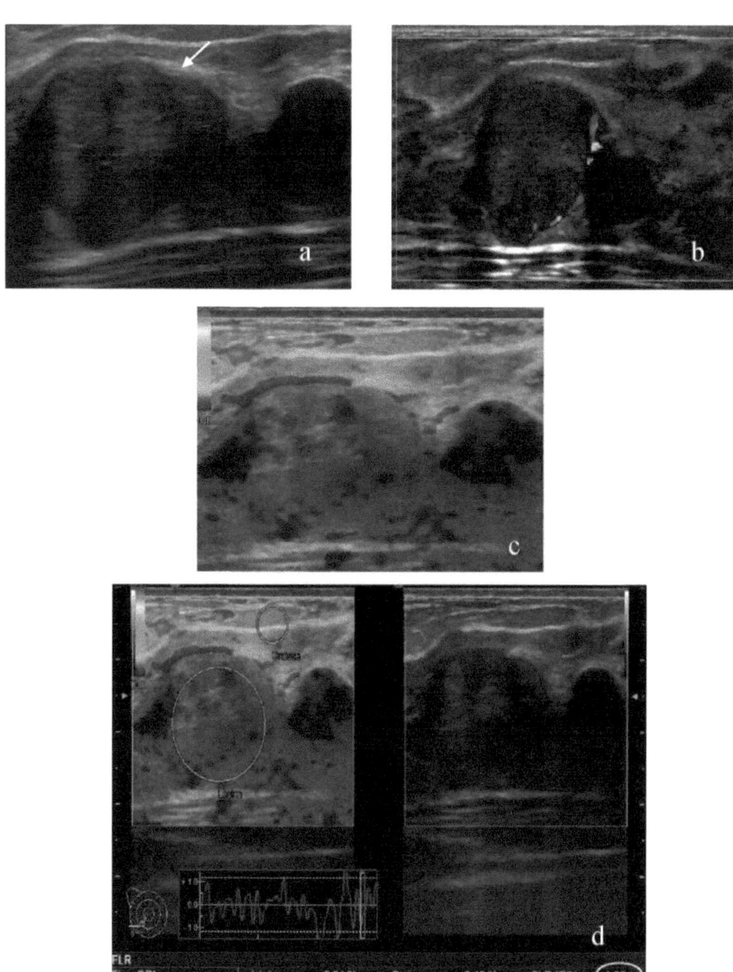

Fig. 23. Cellular fibroadenoma. (a) B-mode ultrasound. Voluminous hypoechoic mass, with macrolobulated contours, homogeneous and horizontal long axis with peripheral pseudocapsule (arrow) (b) Color Doppler. Hypervascularized mass. (c+d) Elastography. Soft mass, elasticity score 2 and elasticity ratio 1.22.

1.5.5. Hyalinized fibroadenoma

Hyalinized fibroadenoma is another variant of fibroadenoma, particularly in post-menopausal women. With age, the mesenchymal component becomes hyalinized, less cellular and more sclerotic (fig. 24). The epithelial component atrophies and calcifications develop as a result of ischemic phenomena, appearing at the periphery of the tumor [49, 50] (fig. 24).

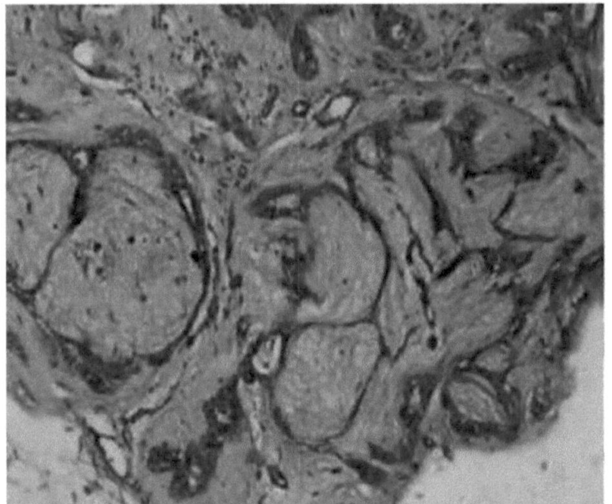

Fig. 24. Hyalinized fibroadenoma. Histology. Hypocellular and sclerotic mesenchymal component. Atrophied epithelial component.

1.5.7.1.Imaging

Mammography is the main imaging technique for diagnosing hyalinized fibroadenomas. It reveals coarse calcifications, initially found in the periphery in the early stages; they then coalesce over time, giving the "popcorn" appearance [50] (figs. 25 and 26 a). The hyalinized fibroadenoma may have a suspicious appearance as an irregular shape, with microlobulated, indistinct or spiculated contours. Hyalinized fibroadenomas have variable density on mammography, most frequently hyperdense secondary to hyalinization and necrosis, degeneration and involutions [50, 51].

On ultrasonography, hyalinized fibroadenomas are generally heterogeneous in echostructure, secondary to hyaline degeneration, irregular in shape and contour, with posterior acoustic attenuation due to the presence of calcifications (fig. 26 b).

Color Doppler cannot differentiate hyalinized fibroadenomas from other fibroadenoma varieties, as lesions are generally avascular (fig. 26 c).

On elastography, hyalinized fibroadenomas are harder than other fibroadenoma variants due to the presence of calcifications (fig. 26 d+e).

MRI of hyalinized fibroadenomas shows different T1 and T2 signals depending on the degree of degeneration. On dynamic sequences, hyalinized fibroadenomas show weak and slow enhancement due to sclera [51].

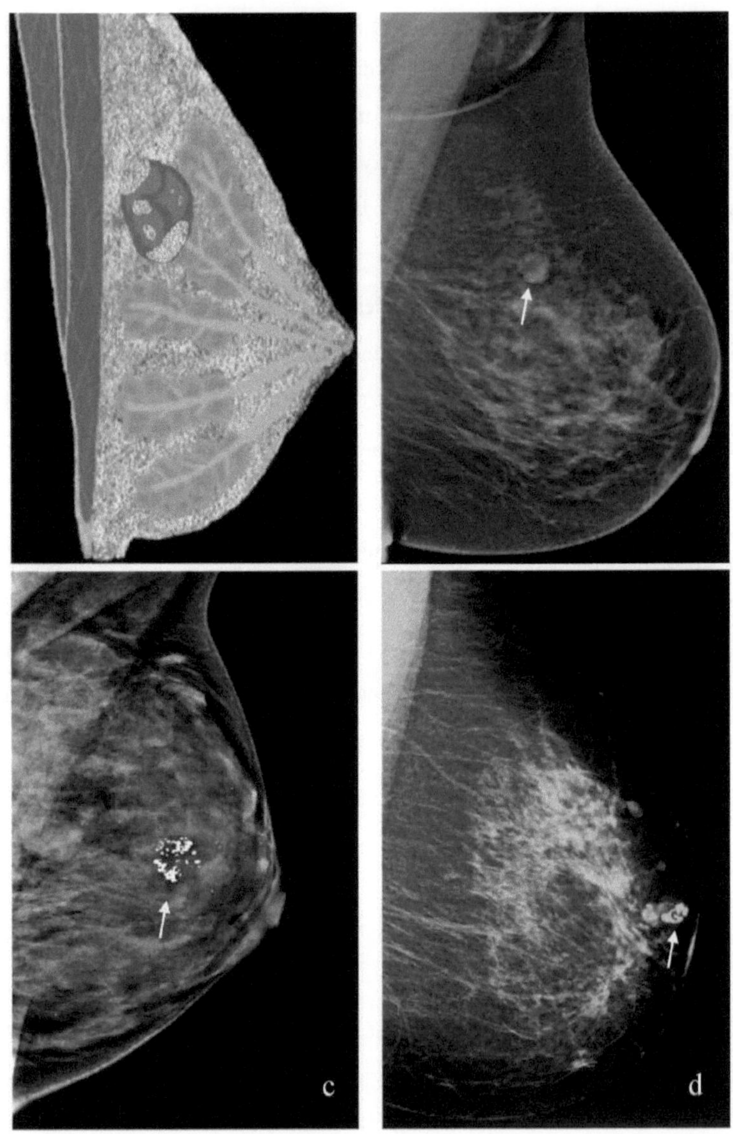

Fig. 25. hyalinized fibroadenoma (a) diagram. (b+c+d) Mammogram. (b) Mass shows peripheral calcifications (arrow). (c+d) Mass shows coarse "popcorn" calcifications (arrows).

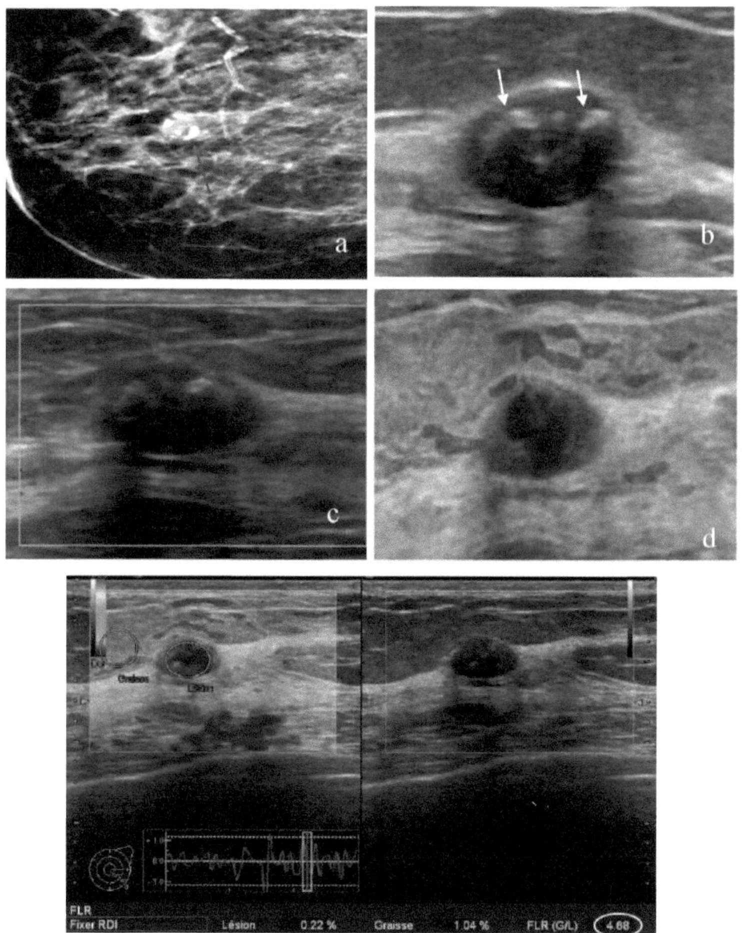

Fig. 26. hyalinized fibroadenoma (a) Mammogram. Isodense mass showing peripheral popcorn calcifications (arrow). (b) B-mode ultrasound. Hypoechoic, circumscribed mass showing calcifications (arrows) (b) Colour Doppler. Non-vascularized mass. (c+d) Elastography. Hard mass, elasticity score 4 and elasticity ratio 4.68.

The different types of fibroadenoma and their imaging are summarized in Table

1.

Tableau 1. Imagerie distinctive des différentes variantes de du fibroadénome.

Fibroadénomes	Spécificité	Mammographie	Échographie	Doppler couleur	Élastographie	IRM
Fibroadénome simple	Caractéristiques classiques Pas d'atypie Pas de mitose	Masse ovale, aux contours circonscrits	Masse ovale, homogène, aux contours circonscrits, isoéchogène, orientation parallèle	Vascularisé (vaisseaux nourriciers, capsulaires, segmentaires)	Masse souple	Septas internes en hyposignal T1, T2, non rehaussés
Fibroadénome juvénile	Adolescente Indolore Croissance rapide	Non nécessaire	Pas de caractéristiques distinctives	Hypervascularisation	Pas de caractéristiques distinctives	Hypersignal T2
Fibroadénome géant	Femme en préménopause Croissance rapide	Similaire au fibroadénome juvénile	Similaire au fibroadénome juvénile	Similaire au fibroadénome juvénile	Pas de caractéristiques distinctives	Similaire au fibroadénome juvénile
Fibroadénome complexe	Histologie : kystes, calcifications épithéliales, adénose sclérosante, métaplasie apocrine Augmente le risque de cancer du sein	Pas de caractéristiques distinctives	Échostructure, hétérogène, forme et contours irréguliers, renforcement, postérieur, kystes et calcifications	Pas de caractéristiques distinctives	Pas de caractéristiques distinctives	Pas de caractéristiques distinctives
Fibroadénome myxoïde	Matrice myxoïde ± associé au syndrome Carney	Pas de caractéristiques distinctives	Important renforcement postérieur	Pas de caractéristiques distinctives	Pas de caractéristiques distinctives	Hypersignal T2, rehaussement rapide et homogène
Fibroadénome cellulaire	Cellularité stromale élevée Problème diagnostique avec les tumeurs phyllodes	Pas de caractéristiques distinctives	Pas de caractéristiques distinctives	Pas de caractéristiques distinctives	Pas de caractéristiques distinctives	Pas de caractéristiques distinctives
Fibroadénome hyalinisé	Femme âgée Faible cellularité stromale et plus de sclérose	Calcifications grossières	Échostructure hétérogène, forme et contours irréguliers, atténuation acoustique postérieure, calcifications	Plus souvent avasculaire	Plus dure que les autres cariantes	Rehaussement faible et lent

1.6. What to do

Several factors need to be taken into account to make the best choice for the management of fibroadenomas, such as the patient's age, family history of breast cancer, symptomatology, size and evolution, but also the physical and psychological discomfort induced.

There are various ways of monitoring and managing the disease: surveillance, surgical or macrobiopsy excision, and ultrasound therapy.

2. Phyllodes tumors

Phyllodes tumours of the breast are rare fibroepithelial tumours, accounting for less than 1% of breast tumours and 2.5% of fibroepithelial tumours. The incidence of phyllodes is low, ranging from 0.3% to 0.9% of all breast tumours [52, 53]. Phyllodes tumours were described by Muller in 1838 under the name cystosarcoma phyllodes. Phyllodes derive from the Latin phyllodium meaning "leaf" [54]. They are a heterogeneous group of tumors with variable prognoses. In 1982, the World Health Organization classified phyllodes tumors into benign, borderline and malignant according to their histopathological characteristics (Table 2) [55]. Benign phyllodes are the most common, accounting for between 35% and 64% of cases, borderline phyllodes for between 7% and 40%, and malignant phyllodes for up to 30% [56, 57]. Phyllodes are difficult to differentiate from other breast tumours prior to surgery. The recurrence rate is 21% for all phyllodes, 10-17% for benign phyllodes, 1425% for borderline phyllodes and 23-30% for malignant phyllodes [58]. Only 2% of phyllodes tumours are metastatic, mainly to lung and bone, rarely to lymph nodes. Virtually only malignant phyllodes tumours can metastasize, about 22% of malignant phyllodes tumours. No metastases are found in borderline or benign phyllodes.

Enlarged lumpectomy with a minimum safety margin of 10 mm for treatment of borderline and benign phyllodes, and mastectomy for malignant phyllodes.

Table 2. WHO classification of phyllodes tumors according to histological features.

Phyllodes tumor/ Histology	Benign	Borderline	Malignant

Degree of stromal hypercellularity	Minime	Moderate	Marked
Nuclear pleomorphism	Minime	Moderate	Marked
Number of mitoses	≤ 4/10 fields at high magnification	5 to 9/10 fields at high magnification	≥ 10/10 fields at high magnification
Tumor margin	Circumscribed	Intermediate	Invasive
Stromal architecture.	Even distribution	Heterogeneous expansion	Marked stromal growth

2.1. Epidemiology and risk factors

Phyllodes tumors can occur at any age, with peak incidence between 30 and 40 years of age. The median age of phyllodes tumors is 45 years, with age ranging from 9 to 93 years [59-62]. It is an exclusively female pathology, with only ten cases reported in the literature of phyllodes tumors in men, often accompanied by gynecomastia [63-65]. The etiology of phyllodes tumours remains unknown, and risk factors have yet to be clearly identified. However, Latin and East Asian women who were born in Central or South America and live in the USA are at higher risk [61, 65-67]. In addition, genetic mutations in chromosomal regions +1q, +5p, +7, +8, 9p, 10p, 6, and 13 correlated with borderline and malignant phyllodes tumors [78]. Few studies have shown the association between family history and phyllodes tumours [69, 70].

Phyllodes tumours mainly affect nulliparous women [71, 72]. Menopausal status remains a matter of debate. Some studies have shown that there is no relationship between phyllodes tumors and the menopausal period. Others suggest that phyllodes tumors are more frequent in genitally active women than in postmenopausal women [73].

On the other hand, several studies have shown that there is a relationship between menopausal status and the degree of malignancy of the tumour. In the study by Kapiris et al [74], 40% of patients with malignant phyllodes were postmenopausal.

2.2. Clinic

In 90% of cases, phyllodes tumors present as a palpable, painless mass. Rapid growth of a known pre-existing mass over several years may suggest the diagnosis of a phyllodes tumor. The phyllodes tumor is usually multilobular and does not adhere to the deep plane. Phyllodes range in size from 0.5 to 30 cm, with an average of 5 to 7.2 cm [75, 76]. Tumor size greater than 3 cm has been correlated with malignancy in several studies [77].

In some cases, bluish discoloration of the skin, ulceration of the skin around the tumour with venous dilatation, nipple retraction and axillary adenopathy may be observed, but these are rare and account for less than 5% of patients [7880].

In conclusion, phyllodes tumors are suspected in the presence of a clinically round, rapidly growing mass $\geq$ 3 cm in size.

2.3. Histology

2.3.1. Macroscopy

Macroscopically, there is nothing to distinguish a phyllodes tumor from a fibroadenoma. It appears as a round or oval mass with circumscribed contours, firm and protruding (fig. 27) [81]. On sectioning, the surface of the mass is beige or pink to grey (fig. 27). Focal nodular extensions can be seen on the surface, between which appear curved fissures giving the "leaf bud" appearance that is more evident in large lesions, as well as haemorrhagic or necrotic areas (fig.27) [81, 82].

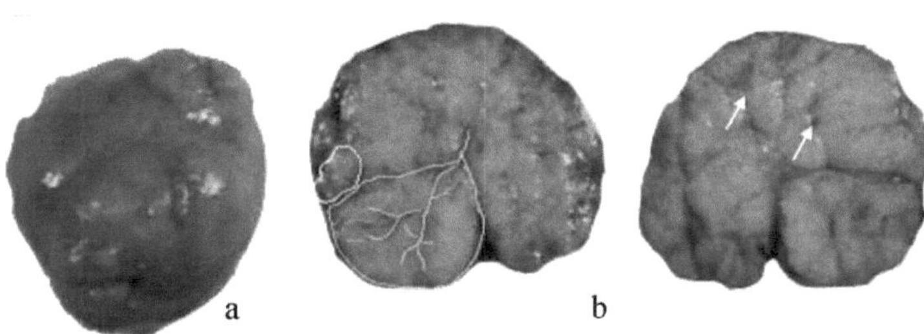

Fig. 27. Phyllodes tumor. (a) Macroscopy. Round, circumscribed mass with lobulated contours, protruding [91]. (b) section slice. Nodular outgrowth (outlined in white. Foliated appearance (outlined in green) with presence of curved slits (arrows) [81].

2.3.2. Microscopy

Microscopically, phyllodes tumors are classified into different grades by the World Health Organization to determine their prognosis and clinical behavior [55]. These include benign, borderline and malignant phyllodes according to histological criteria, including stromal cellularity, degree of nuclear pleomorphism, mitotic activity, tumor margin and stromal architecture (Table 2) [55]. Benign phyllodes tumours account for 35% to 64% of cases, while the malignant form represents around 25% of cases [56, 57, 83]. In benign phyllodes tumors (grade I tumors), the mesenchymal component is characterized by minimal hypercellularity, with monomorphic nuclei, showing rare mitoses of less than 5/10 fields at high magnification [84] (fig. 28). Depending on the degree of nuclear atypia and mitotic activity of the connective tissue component, borderline phyllodes or grade II tumors are characterized by moderate nuclear irregularities, mitoses between 5 and 9/10 fields at high magnification, and malignant phyllodes or grade III tumors correspond to a sarcoma, with a predominant connective tissue component, marked nuclear irregularities and mitoses greater than 10/10 fields at high magnification [85]. The heterogeneity of the mesenchymal component may give rise to foci of metaplasia (osteochondral, fatty).

The epithelial component, consisting of a double layer of epithelial and myoepithelial cells, takes the form of stretched canals, located opposite the clefts, with a peripheral distribution known as splayed, taking on a foliaceous appearance, hence the name phyllodes, derived from the Latin "phyllodium" and the Greek "phyllodes". This component may be the site of simple ductal hyperplasia or cylindrical metaplasia.

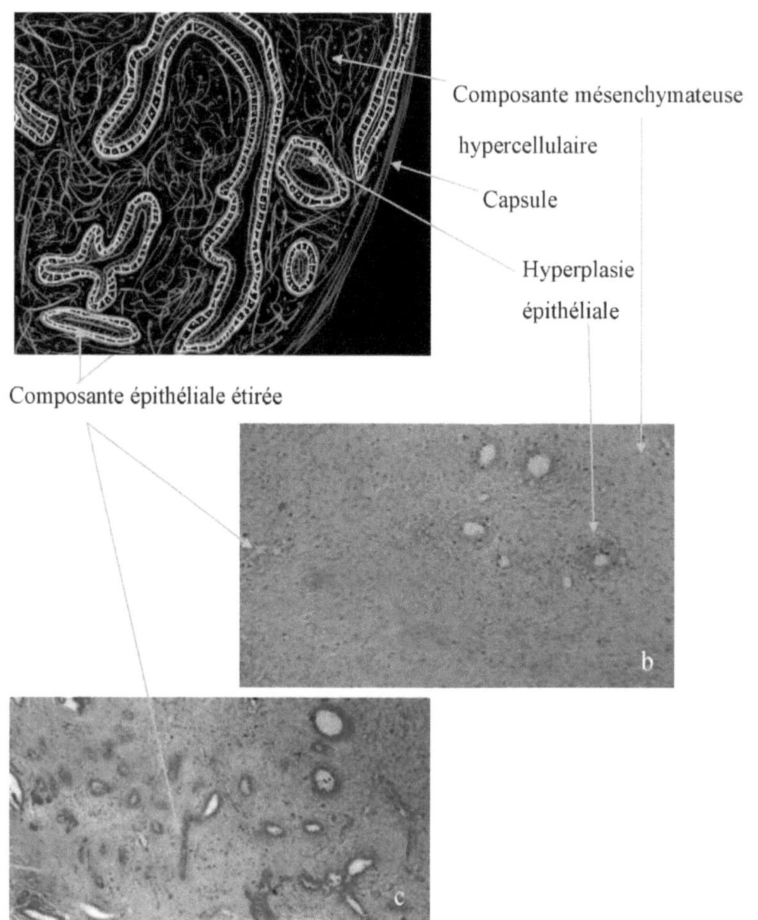

Fig. 28. Phyllodes tumor. Microscopy. (a) Schematic diagram. (b+c). Histology.

2.4. Imaging

2.4.1. Mammography

Mammographic findings are non-specific, and do not provide a reliable preoperative diagnosis. Clinical characteristics, tumor growth rate and patient age must also be taken into consideration.

The phyllodes tumor may appear as an oval or round mass, with circumscribed or lobulated contours, iso or more often hyperdense [65, 86] (fig. 29). Non-circumscribed contours may be found in malignant phyllodes.

Calcifications are rare due to their rapid growth, but can be observed in cases of necrosis and when present, are coarse similar to those of a fibroadenoma. Despite the overlapping mammographic features of benign and malignant phyllodes, the literature suggests that a size greater than 3 cm should raise the possibility of a malignant phyllodes tumour [87].

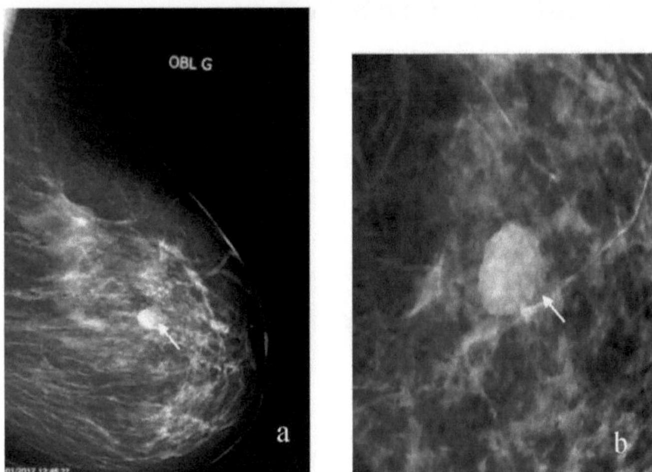

Fig. 29. Phyllodes tumor: (a) Mammogram; (b) magnification.
Oval, lobulated mass, hyperdense (arrows).

2.4.2. B-mode ultrasound

Phyllodes tumors present as oval or oral masses with circumscribed contours [88, 89]. The internal echostructure is variable, usually homogeneous hypoechoic or heterogeneous, with cystic zones associated with haemorrhagic or necrotic areas, as well as the presence of liquid fissures corresponding to stretched ductal structures, suggestive of a phyllodes tumour [88-90] (fig. 30). The high stromal cellularity of these tumours generally results in posterior enhancement [90] (fig.

30).

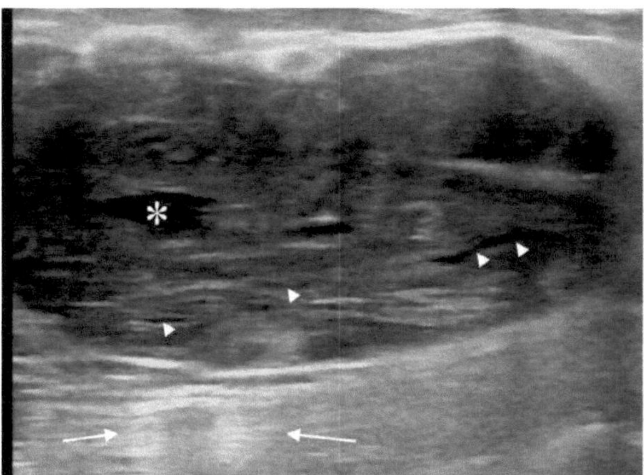

Fig. 30. Phyllodes tumor. Ultrasonography. Oval mass, with macrolobulated contours, hypoechoic, orientation parallel to the skin, heterogeneous by the presence of anechoic cystic areas (asterisk), as well as fluidic fissures (arrowheads), posterior acoustic enhancement (arrows).

2.4.3. Color Doppler

Phyllodes tumors are often highly vascularized on color Doppler, with both central and peripheral vascularization [91, 92] (fig.31).

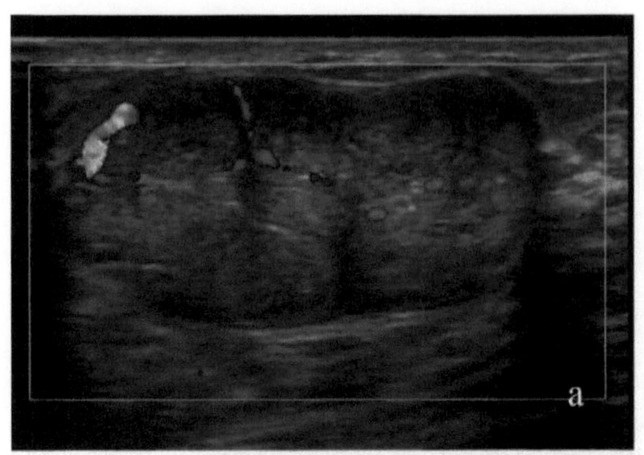

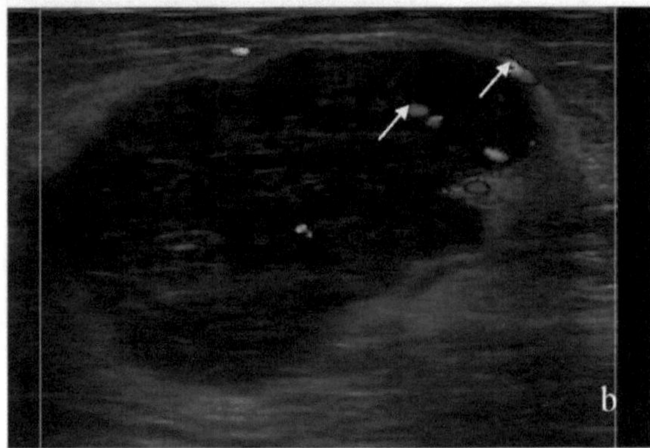

Fig. 31. Phyllodes tumors. Color Doppler. Hypervascularization (arrows). (a) Mass in a 21-year-old woman. (b) Mass in a 40-year-old woman.

2.4.4. Elastography

Elastography of phyllodes tumors is more discriminating than B-mode ultrasonography, most often showing a cocoon-like appearance with a soft center and harder periphery of Itoh score 3 [93] (fig.32).

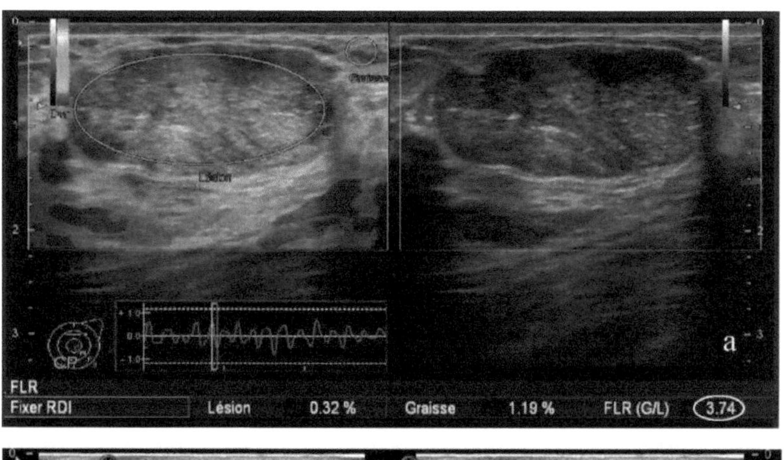

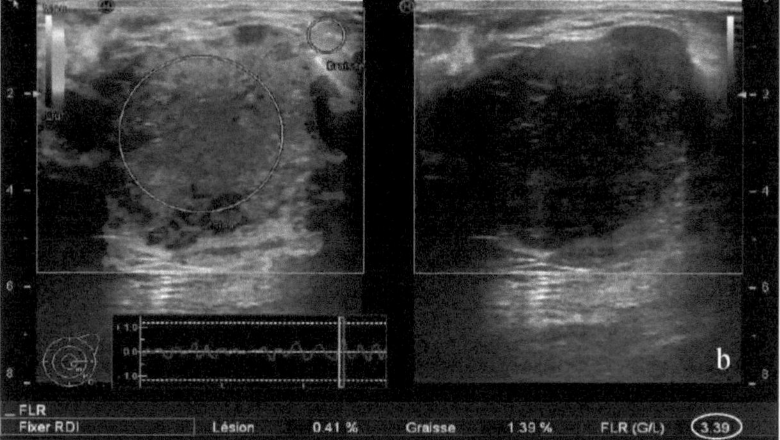

Fig. 32. Phyllodes tumors. Elastography. (a) Phyllodes tumor in a 21-year-old woman, intermediate hardness, elasticity score 3 and estimated elasticity ratio 3.74. (b) Phyllodes tumor in a 40-year-old woman, intermediate hardness, elasticity score 3 and estimated elasticity ratio 3.39.

2.4.3. MRI

Although magnetic resonance imaging (MRI) is extremely sensitive for the detection of breast cancer, it is still difficult to differentiate phyllodes tumours from other types of breast tumour [94, 95]. On MRI, phyllodes tumors appear as an oval, round or lobulated mass with circumscribed contours, in hyposignal on T1-weighted sequences, although the presence of an intratumoral hemorrhagic component leads to signal enhancement, in T2 hypersignal and STIR, with signal intensity on T2 sequences of the tumor less than or equal to the signal of normal breast parenchyma. On T2 sequences, liquid intralesional fissures may be observed in hypersignal, more frequent in benign tumours than in borderline or malignant tumours [96, 97] (fig. 33). Phyllodes tumors that are hypersignal on diffusion sequences with low ADC more often suggest a borderline or malignant phyllodes tumor, as evidenced histologically by stromal hypercellularity [98].

On sequences after contrast injection, all three types of enhancement can be seen in phyllodes. Kinetic criteria do not appear to be discriminating in determining the histological grade of phyllodes tumors [99, 100].

With regard to the spectroscopy sequence, several studies have shown that spectroscopy cannot differentiate benign from borderline and malignant phyllodes [98, 101].

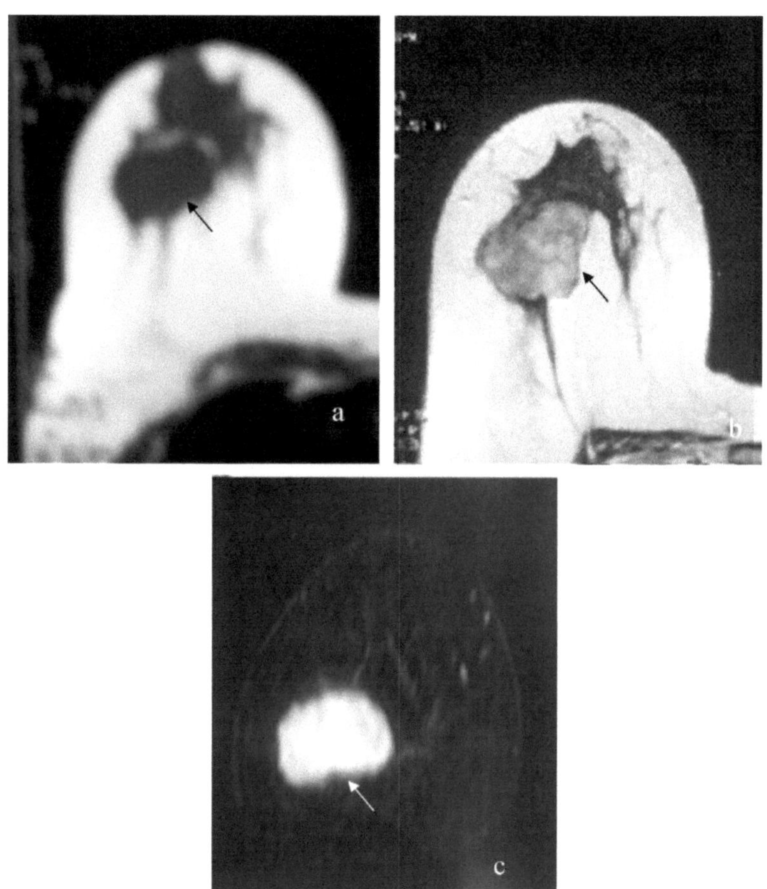

Fig. 33. Phyllodes tumor. MRI (a) T1 sequence. (b) T2 sequence. (c) Subtracted injected T1 sequence. Roughly rounded mass with lobulated contours, hyposignal T1, hypersignal T2, enhanced after injection of contrast medium (arrows).

2.5. What to do

Treatment is surgical: enlarged lumpectomy with a 10 mm resection margin for benign and borderline phyllodes, mastectomy for malignant tumours.

Enucleation is not recommended, as there is a risk of recurrence.

3. Papilloma

Papilloma is a lesion with intracanal development, in the lumen of a large proximal retroareolar galactophoric duct, often a single lesion, or in a distal duct, often multiple lesions.

3.1. Epidemiology

They account for 1-2% of all breast tumours. The age of onset is between 30 and 40 years [102]. It is located in the main ducts, and usually measures between 3 and 10 mm [103].

3.2. Clinic

A single papilloma is usually revealed by a unilateral unipore discharge, spontaneous or induced, either serous or bloody, associated or not with a palpable mass.

3.3. Histology

Papillomas are characterized microscopically by papillae consisting of a conjunctivo-vascular axis bordered by a double bed of myoepithelial and epithelial cells. The epithelial component may be simple hyperplasia or apocrine metaplasia [104] (fig. 34).

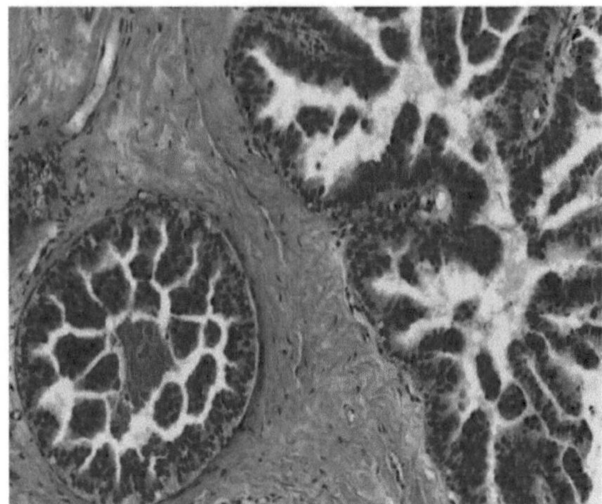

Fig. 34. Papilloma. Microscopy. Often multiple, located more peripherally in the ductal system, and characterized by arborized connective axes bordered by two epithelial and myoepithelial cell layers [105].

3.4. Imaging

Papillomas often do not translate mammographically and should be investigated by galactography [106, 107]. Dense, irregular calcifications may be visible, secondary to ischemic phenomena [108, 109]. On ultrasonography, the papilloma may be visible as one or more echogenic, homogeneous masses, with more or less circumscribed contours, within a ductal ectasia [108, 109]. In the case of galactophoric dilatation, it produces an image of intracystic vegetation [110] (fig. 35). More rarely, it presents as a solid mass on imaging [111], and is diagnosed on biopsy [107] (fig. 36).

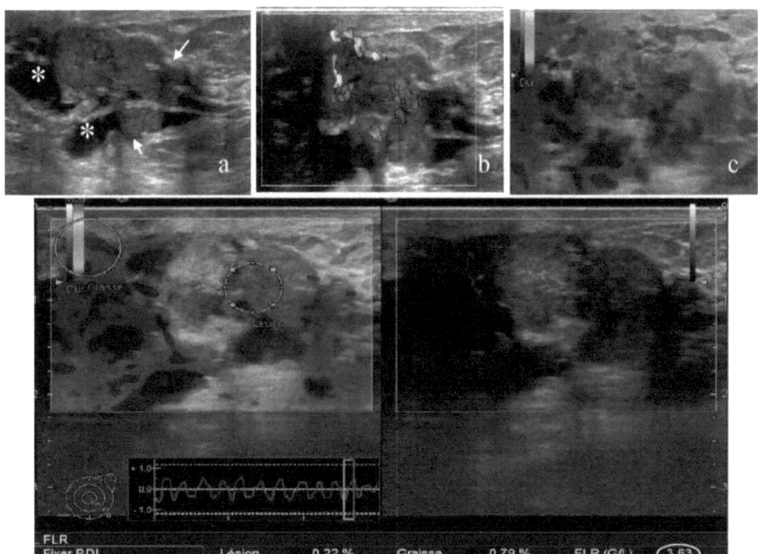

Fig. 35. Papilloma. (a) B-mode ultrasound. Echogenic masses (arrows), seated in an anechogenic dilated duct (asterisks). (b) Color Doppler. Hypervascularized masses. (c+d) Elastography. The largest mass was of intermediate hardness, with an elasticity score of 2 and an elasticity ratio of 3.63.

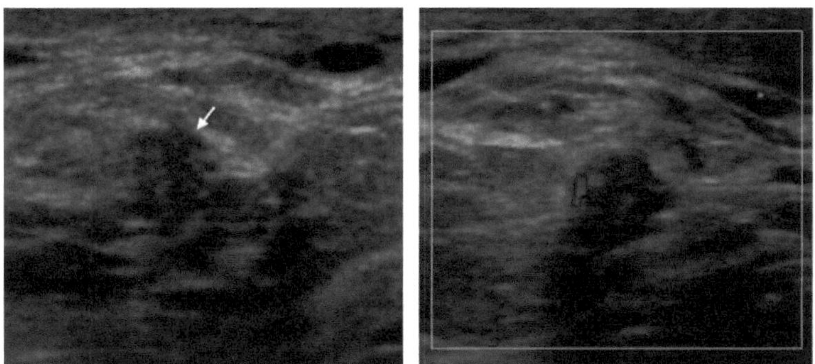

Fig. 36. Papilloma. (a) B-mode ultrasound. Hypoechoic masses with microlobulated contours (arrow), (b) color Doppler. Masses show peripheral vascularization.

3.4. What to do

Because of the risk of degeneration, which is greater for the distal form (10-30%), and of underestimation of papillary cancer at biopsy, with a false-negative rate of 10-20%, surgical excision is the rule [112-114].

In the case of papillomas smaller than 15 mm, excision by macrobiopsy under suction is feasible [115]. In the case of multiple papillomas, because of their extension, segmentectomy is often performed.

4. Adenomyepithelioma

Adenomyepithelioma is a very rare tumour. Its incidence is therefore unknown, with only 4 comprehensive studies and occasional cases reported in the literature, around 150 cases [116].

4.1. Histology

This benign lesion is characterized by a proliferation of both myoepithelial cells and differentiated epithelial cells.

The nosology of this lesion is controversial, both radio-clinically and anatomopathologically. In most cases, it evolves in a benign mode with an aggressive potential characterized by multiple recurrences; exceptionally, it evolves in a malignant mode with metastases, which explains why some authors classify it as a myoepithelial tumor, while others classify it as a rare mammary carcinoma [117].

4.2. Imaging

On mammography, the tumor appears as an isodense, well-circumscribed mass (fig. 37).

On ultrasonography, adenomyepithelioma often appears as a circumscribed mass, sometimes with macrolobulated contours. Its echostructure is hypoechoic, heterogeneous and associated with microcystic changes [118-123] (fig. 37).

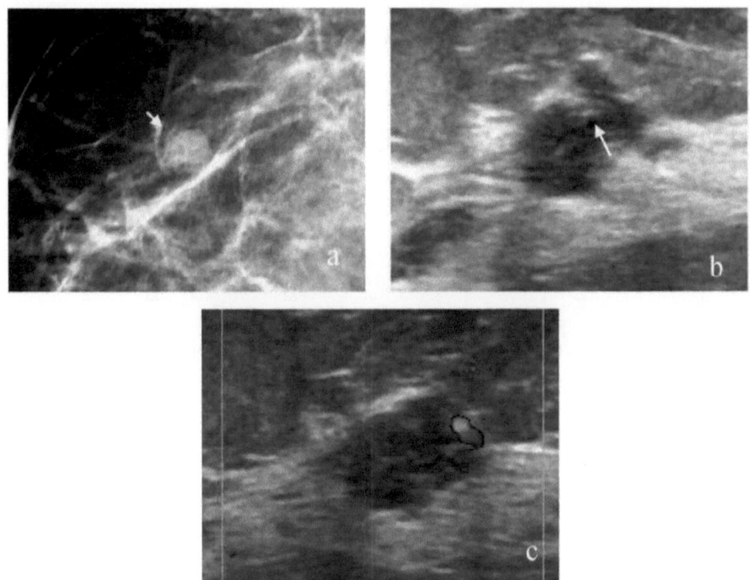

Fig. 37. Adenomyepithelioma (a) Mammogram. Oval-shaped, macrolobulated, isodense mass (arrow). (b) B-mode ultrasound. Mass with macrolobulated contours, hypoechoic, heterogeneous with microcystic remodelling (arrow). (c) Color Doppler. Peripherally vascularized mass.

4.3. What to do

The lesion is considered a benign tumor, but due to some cases of local and distant recurrence, surgery with a healthy margin is recommended.

5. Pseudoangiomatous stromal hyperplasia *(PASH)*

Better known as PASH (Pseudo-Angiomatous Stromal Hyperplasia). PASH is a rare benign mesenchymal lesion, first described by Vuitch, et al. in 1986 [124]. Only around 100 cases have been reported in the literature [125]. It consists of a proliferation of benign myofibroblastic cells. Described at any age, but mainly in premenopausal women, with an average age of 40 [124, 125]. It can be seen in postmenopausal women, particularly those receiving hormone replacement therapy, but can also be encountered in men, particularly those with gynecomastia. PASH appears to be caused by hormonal imbalances [125, 126].

This tumor is often discovered by chance, during histological examination of a breast lesion [127-129]. It is quite common, but often goes unnoticed. In the study by Ibrahim et al [130], among 200 cases of mastectomy and biopsy, microscopic foci of PASH were found in 23% of cases.

The clinical presentation of PASH varies. It may appear as a palpable mass with a firm, mobile consistency, mimicking a benign lesion [129, 131]. Rarely, it may develop very rapidly, rapidly increasing breast volume with diffuse thickening or even an orange peel appearance, mimicking a cancerous lesion [127].

5.1. Histology

5.1.1. Macroscopy

Macroscopically, in nodular forms, the mass is well-limited with a clear outer surface, sometimes surrounded by a pseudocapsule, varying in size from 1 to 18 cm, grayish-white in color, homogeneous and firm in consistency. In some cases, it contains a few cystic cavities without necrotic or haemorrhagic areas, mimicking a fibroadenoma [124, 125, 127, 132]. In diffuse forms, the surgical specimen contains no macroscopically detectable mass [132].

5.1.2. Microscopy

Microscopically, PASH is characterized by an excess of collagenous connective tissue due to proliferation of myofibroblastic cells, in which ductal and lobular epithelial structures are normal but scattered. The dense connective tissue forms a complex network of optically empty, anastomosing pseudovascular slits. These slits are lined solely by flattened, spindle-shaped myofibroblastic cells without atypia or mitosis, sometimes showing a concentric arrangement around the lobules [124, 125, 127, 132]. The term "pseudoangiomatous" has been proposed to emphasize its peculiar histological appearance mimicking vascular proliferation (fig. 38). This often poses a diagnostic problem with low-grade angiosarcoma, which is formed by vascular clefts bordered by vascular spindle cell endothelium [124, 125]. Formal differentiation between the two lesions is made by immunohistochemical study of the cells lining the clefts. In angiosarcoma, the immunohistochemical study shows positivity for the vascular markers CD31 and factor VIII [131]. In contrast to PASH, endothelial cell markers are negative but positive for vimentin, anti-smooth muscle Ac, CD34 and progesterone receptors [131].

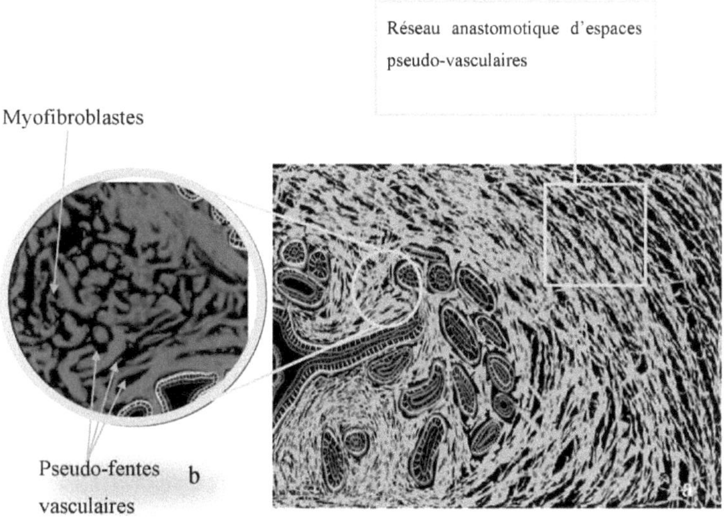

Fig. 38. PASH. Microscopy. (a) Diagram. Network of anastomosing fissures within the inter- and intra-lobular fibro-hyaline stroma. (b) Enlarged diagram. Proliferation of myofibroblastic cells with vascular pseudoclefts.

5.2. Imaging

Mammographic findings range from a focal asymmetry of density to an oval or round mass, usually circumscribed, dense, homogeneous and free of calcification [133, 134].

On ultrasonography, in the nodular form, PASH appears as a mass, oval in shape, with circumscribed contours, long horizontal axis parallel to the skin, hypoechoic, of discreetly heterogeneous echostructure with the presence of a microcystic component [134] (fig. 39). The PASH shows little or no vascularity on color Doppler and is soft on elastography (figs. 40 and 41). On MRI, PASH enhances after contrast injection.

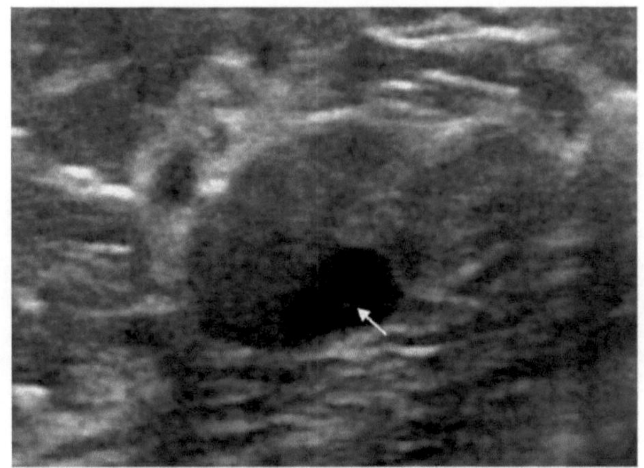

Fig. 39. PASH. Ultrasound scan. Circumscribed oval-shaped mass with large horizontal axis, more or less homogeneous echostructure with microcystic component (arrow).

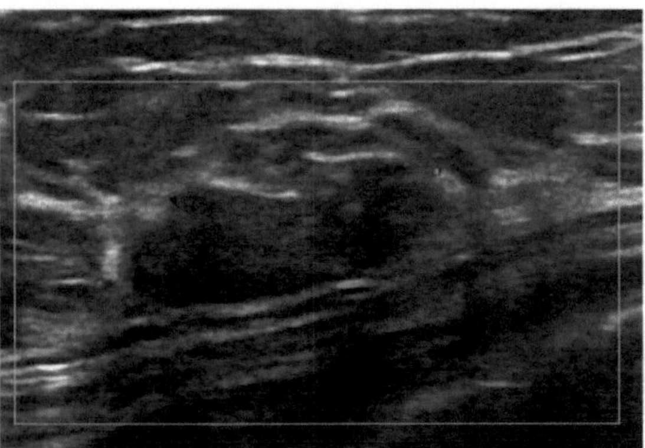

Fig. 40 PASH. Color Doppler. Non-vascularized mass.

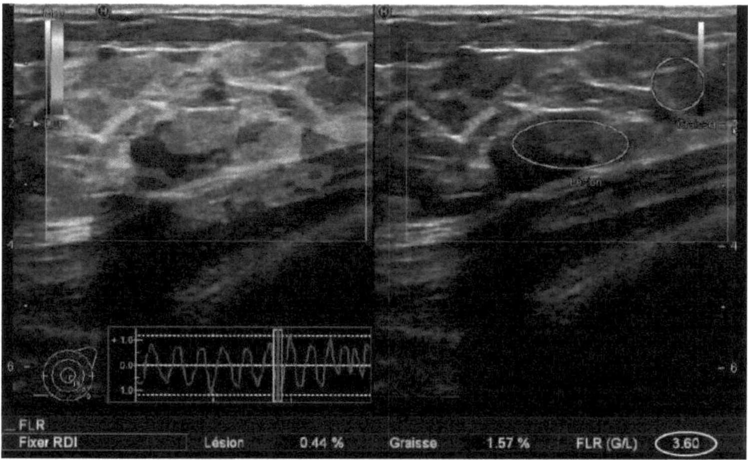

Fig. 41. PASH. Elastography. Soft mass, elasticity score 2 and estimated elasticity ratio 3.6.

5.3. What to do

Treatment consists of complete surgical excision, with healthy histological margins and subsequent surveillance, due to the risk of recurrence, which is frequent in the first three years in up to 20% of cases [75].

6. Hamartome

The hamartoma corresponds to normal breast tissue of anarchic distribution. It is a rare benign lesion of the breast, representing around 4.8% of all benign lesions [135], and was first described in 1971 by Arrigoni et al [136]. The hamartoma comprises a variable amount of glandular, fibrous and fatty tissue [137]. This tumour occurs at any age from puberty onwards, most often in premenopausal women [138, 139]. Diagnosis is often made on mammography [140]. Histological and radiological aspects are variable and depend on its fatty tissue content [137]. It is most often asymptomatic, but may be palpable if bulky, or when the fibro-glandular component is predominant.

Identification of these lesions avoids the need for systematic surgical excision on the one hand and, on the other, prevents the development of breast cancer in these normally benign tumors [140].

6.1. Histology

6.1.1. Macroscopy

Macroscopically, the tumor is round or oval in shape, well limited and sometimes lobulated, surrounded by a thin fibrous pseudocapsule. The section slice shows either a homogeneous whitish fibro-glandular appearance resembling a fibroadenoma; a yellowish appearance resembling a lipoma; or a mixed heterogeneous appearance [81, 141, 142].

6.1.2. Microscopy

Microscopy reveals normal breast tissue: fibro-glandular and adipose tissue in varying proportions. Fibrocystic changes are common, but epithelial hyperplasia is rare in most series [135, 143, 144]. However, one series reported ductal hyperplasia in 27% and coexistence with fibroadenomas in 12% [145]. Only a few cases of carcinoma in situ and infiltrating carcinoma developed in a hamartoma have been described [146-149].

6.2. Imaging

On imaging, the mammographic appearance of the hamartoma is described as a "breast in the breast", and a double-component appearance - clear, which is the fatty component, and dense, which corresponds to the fibro-glandular tissue, delimited by a thin capsule - is pathognomonic [150-152] (fig. 42). When it is small or the fatty component is in the minority, its appearance mimics that of a benign tumour [150, 153]. In dense breasts, the hamartoma appears as a focal asymmetry of density, without visualization of the pseudocapsule, and will be difficult to diagnose [154].

On ultrasonography, the two tissue components form a heterogeneous mass with nodular areas that are isoechoic with fat and hyperechoic with normal glandular tissue; the capsule is rarely perceptible (fig. 43). On color Doppler, the vascularity of the hamartoma is identical to that of the normal mammary gland (fig. 44). The mass is very soft on elastography, almost the same hardness as subcutaneous fat [150, 152, 155-157] (fig. 45).

On MRI, the fatty component, visible on morphological sequences as a T1, T2 hypersignal, with a drop in signal on fat saturation sequences. After contrast injection, the fibroglandular component of the hamartoma enhances in the same way as the adjacent mammary parenchyma, sometimes slightly more, but without kinetics of pejorative enhancement or wash-out [149, 158, 159].

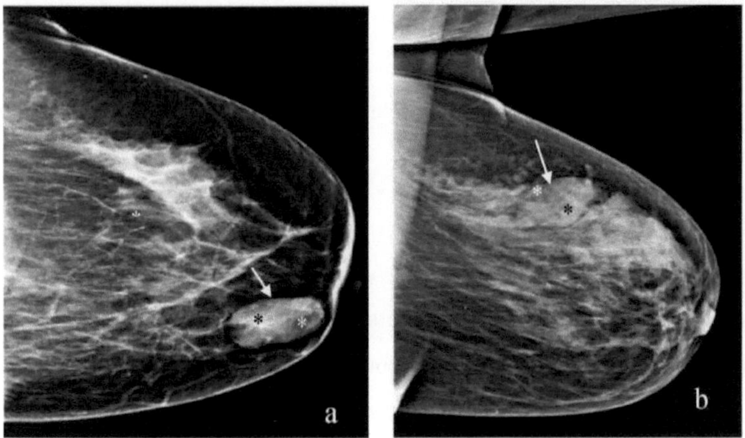

Fig. 42. Hamartoma. Mammogram (a) frontal view (b) oblique view.
Circumscribed, oval mass of the QSI, with a double component: light (fat) (white
asterisk) and dense (fibroglandular tissue) (black asterisk), delimited by a thin
capsule (arrow).

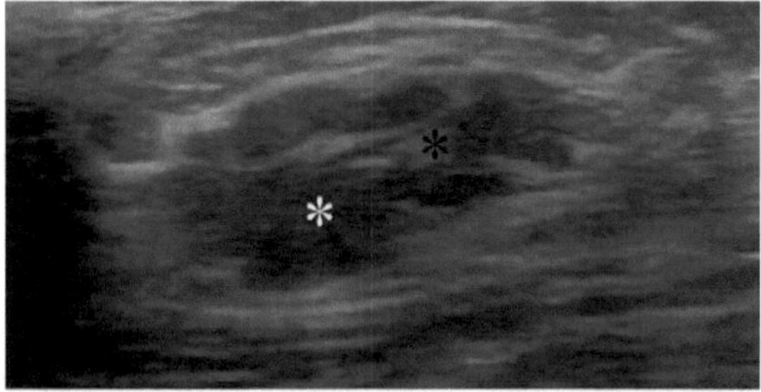

Fig. 43. Hamartoma. Ultrasound. Mass of mixed echostructure, hypoechoic but
isoechoic to fat (white asterisk) and hyperechoic but isoechoic to normal mammary
gland (black asterisk). Note that the capsule cannot be individualized.

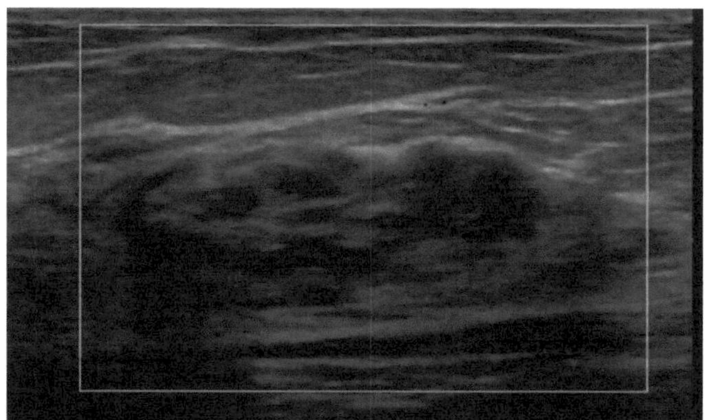

Fig. 44. Hamartoma. Color Doppler. Avascular mass.

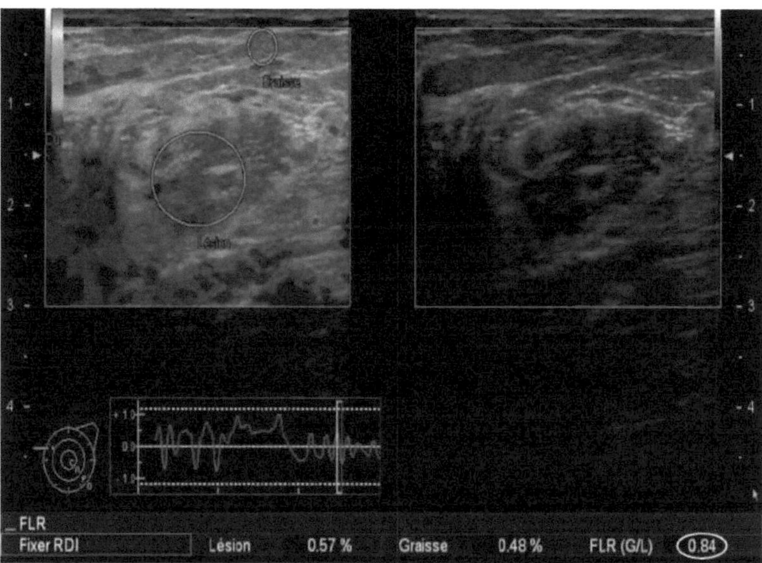

Fig. 45. Hamartoma. Elastography. Very soft mass, elasticity score 1 and elasticity ratio estimated at 0.84, virtually the same hardness as subcutaneous fat.

6.3. What to do

No follow-up or management is recommended for hamartomas [160]. Surgical removal is indicated in cases of discomfort or deformity of the mammary gland [160]. Malignant transformation of hamartomas is very rare [146-149]. The rare cases of carcinoma in situ or infiltrating carcinoma in hamartomas must be treated as a cancerous lesion.

7. Rarer benign tumors

7.1. Amyloid tumors [161, 162]

They are exceptional. They present as a palpable, firm, ill-defined mass. Mammography may show a large, aspecific mass. Ultrasound reveals a mass with circumscribed, sometimes irregular contours. Its echostructure is heterogeneous, combining hypo- and hyperechoic areas, with partial posterior attenuation opposite the most echogenic zones. Amyloid tumors may recur after biopsy and excision.

7.2. Lactating adenoma

Lactating adenoma is a benign lesion, occurring during pregnancy or postpartum. Its true nature is controversial. Some authors suggest that it is a variant of fibroadenoma, tubular adenoma or lobular hyperplasia with pregnancy-related changes. Histologically, it is a well-circumscribed lobular proliferation consisting of a compact aggregate of lobules and secretory hyperplasia. Characteristically, it regresses spontaneously. It may undergo necrotic and inflammatory changes.

7.2.1. Imaging

On mammography, a lactating adenoma is usually seen as a fibroadenoma-like mass, oval in shape, with its long axis parallel to the skin and regular contours. On ultrasound, the lesion is heterogeneous (Fig. 46). In some cases, there are fatty areas within it, suggestive of the diagnosis, radiolucent on mammography and echogenic on ultrasound. These areas correspond to the milk fat secreted by hyperplasia. In some cases, it may present more equivocal aspects, particularly in cases of necrosis [163-165]

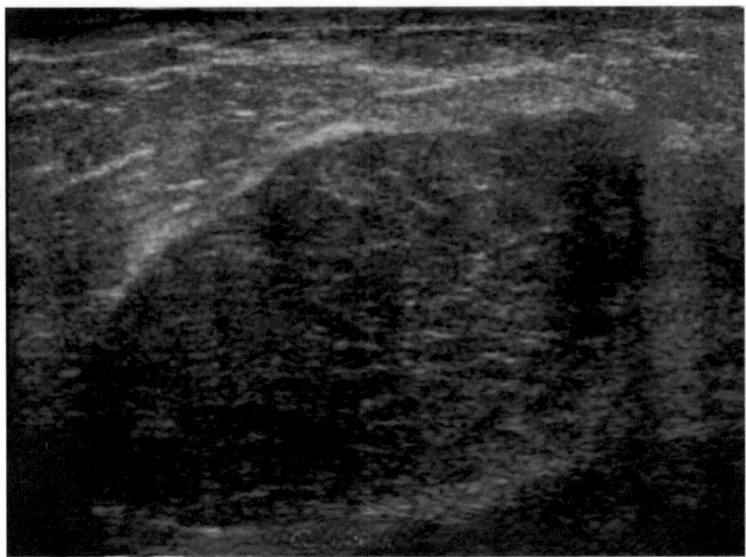

Fig. 46. Lactating adenoma. Ultrasound mode B. Heterogeneous hypoechoic mass with discreetly indistinct contours in a pregnant woman.

7.3. Juvenile papillomatosis

It is a rare pathology of adolescents and young women, described histologically in 1980 by Rosen et al [166] and ultrasonographically by Kersschot et al [167].

7.3.1. Histology

It associates lesions of florid epithelial hyperplasia, sometimes atypical, and microcystic lesions with papillary and apocrine metaplastic epithelial coating.

7.3.2. Clinic

The tumor is often palpable, firm, mobile, nonspecific but painful, discovered in a young woman usually between the ages of 15 and 35. A family history of breast cancer is common [168]. Breast cancer may also be present at the time of discovery.

7.3.3. Imaging

Mammography reveals a rounded or oval mass with lobulated contours. Microcalcifications may be associated [169].

On ultrasonography, a circumscribed or macrolobulated, double-component, solid mass is seen, with microcystic remodelling predominating in the peripheral part of the mass [170] (fig. 47). More rarely, the mass may appear poorly defined, heterogeneous and suspicious of malignancy.

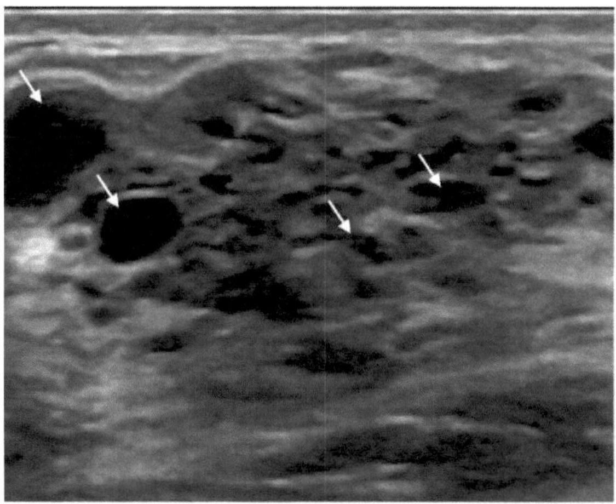

Fig. 47. Juvenile papillomatosis. Complex mass of multiple microcysts (arrows) [171].

7.3.4. What to do

Surgical excision is recommended as a preventive measure, due to the high risk of breast cancer. This lesion is thought to be a phenotypic marker of genetic predisposition to breast cancer [172].

References

1. Couturaud B, Fitoussi A. Anatomy/surgery of breast cancer. Conservative treatment, oncoplasty. Techniques chirurgicales gynécologie. Elsevier Masson; 2011; 4-7.

2. Chu B, Crystal P. Imaging of fibroepithelial lesions: a pictorial essay. Can Assoc Radiol J 2012;63:135-145.

3. Hughes, L., Mansel, R., & Webster, D. T. (1987). Aberrations of normal development and involution (ANDI): a new perspective on pathogenesis and nomenclature of benign breast disorders. The Lancet, 330 (8571), 1316-1319.

4. Tavassoli FA Pathology of the breast, 2nd edn. Appleton & Lange, Stamford, CT, 1999.

5. Goehring C and Morabia A. Epidemiology of benign breast disease, with special attention to histologic types. Epidemiologic reviews, 1997, vol. 19, no 2, p. 310327.

6. Felecia Cerrato and Brian I. Labow. Diagnosis and management of fibroadenomas in the adolescent breast. Seminars in Plastic Surgery, vol. 27, no. 1, February 2013,

7. Noguchi S., Motomura K., Inaji N. and Imaoka S. Clonal analysis of fibroadenoma and phyllodes tumor of the breast. Cancer Research, vol. 53, no 17, 1993.

8. Greenberg R., Skornick Y. and Kaplan O. *Management of breast fibroadenomas.* Journal of General Internal Medicine, vol. 13, n° 9, 1998, p. 640645

9. Maleeha Ajmal, Myra Khan and Kelly Van F ossen, Stat Pearls, Stat Pearls Publishing, 2021.

10. Robert A Philibert and Anup Madan. Role of MED12 in transcription and

human behavior. Pharmacogenomics, vol. 8, no 8, 2007.

11. Michelle Lee and Hooman T Soltanian. Breast fibroadenomas in adolescents: current perspectives. Adolescent Health, Medicine and Therapeutics, vol. 6, 2015.

12. Courtillot C, Plu-Bureau G, Binart N, Balleyguier C, Sigal-Zafrani B, Goffin V, Kuttenn F, Kelly PA, Touraine P. Benign breast diseases. J Mammary Gland Biol Neoplasia. 2005 Oct;10(4):325-35.

13. Dent DM, Cant PJ. Fibroadenoma. World J Surg. 1989 Nov-Dec;13(6):706-10.

14. Ajmal M, Khan M, Van Fossen K. Breast Fibroadenoma. 2022.

15. Herin M. Atlas pathologie générale. 2002 ; p 67.

16. Oluwole SF, Freeman HP. Analysis of benign breast lesions in blacks. Am. J. Surg. June 1979;137.

17. Krings G, Bean GR, Chen YY. Fibroepithelial lesions; the WHO spectrum. Semin Diagn Pathol 2017;34:438-52.

18. Stavros AT. Benign solid nodules: specific pathologic diagnoses. In: Stavros AT, editor. Breast ultrasound. Philadelphia: Lippincott Williams & Wilkins; 2004. p. 528-96.

19. Cole-Beuglet C, Soriano R, Kurtz AB, et al. Ultrasound, x-ray mammography and histopathology of cystosarcoma phylloides. Radiology 1983;146:481-6.

20. Strano S, Gombos EC, Friedland O, et al. Color Doppler imaging of fibroadenomas of the breast with histopathologic correlation. J Clin Ultrasound 2004;32:317-22.

21. Hochman MG, Orel SG, Powell CM, et al. Fibroadenomas: variety of MR appearances with radiologic-histopathologic correlation. Radiology 1997;204: 1239.

22. Davis S, Wallace A. A 19 year old with complete androgen insensitivity syndrome and juvenile fibroadenoma of the breast. Breast J 2001;7:430-3.

23. Chung EM, Cube R, Hall GJ, et al. From the archives of the AFIP: breast masses in children and adolescents: radiologic-pathologic correlation. Radiographics 2009; 29:907-31.

24. AbdelHadi M. Giant juvenile fibroadenoma: experience from a university hospital. J Family Community Med 2005;12:91-5. https://doi.org/10.1055/s-0033-1343992.

25. Virginie Grouthier. Prospective follow-up of 60 women with breast polyadenomatosis: radiological description and factors associated with its evolution. Human Medicine and Pathology. 2015. dumas-01223448.

26. Chu B, Crystal P. Imaging of fibroepithelial lesions: a pictorial essay. Can Assoc Radiol J. 2012 May;63(2):135-45.

27. Cerrato F, Labow BI. Diagnosis and management of fibroadenomas in the adolescent breast. Semin Plast Surg 2013;27:23-5. https://doi.org/10.1055/s-0033- 1343992.

28. Mendelson EB, Bohm-Velez M, Berg WA, et al. ACR BI-RADS atlas, breast imaging reporting and data system. Reston (VA): American College of Radiology; 2013.

29. Kim SJ, Park YM, Jung SJ, et al. Sonographic appearances of juvenile fibroadenoma of the breast. J Ultrasound Med 2014;33:1879-84.

30. Baxi M, Agarwal A, Mishra A, et al. Multiple bilateral giant juvenile fibroadenomas of breast. Eur J Surg 2000;166:828-30.

31. Hanna RM, Ashebu SD. Giant fibroadenoma of the breast in an Arab population.
Australas Radiol 2002;46:252-6. https://doi.org/10.1046zj.1440-1673.2002.01054.x.

32. Sharma S, Rana BP. Giant fibroadenoma of breast: a diagnostic dilemma in a middle aged woman. Adv Cytol Pathol 2017;2:109-12.

33. Arowolo OA, Akinkuolie AA, Adisa AO, et al. Giant fibroadenoma presenting

like fungating breast cancer in a Nigerian teenager. Afr Health Sci 2013;13:162-5.

34. Dupont WD, Page DL, Parl FF et al. Long-term risk of breast cancer in women with fibroadenoma. The New England Journal of Medicine. 1994 ; 331 :10-5.

35. Kuiper A, Mommers EM, Wall E, et al. Histopathology of fibroadenoma of the breast. Am J Clin Pathol 2001;115:736-42.

36. Dupont WD, Page DL, Parl FF, et al. Long-term risk of breast cancer in women with fibroadenoma. N Engl J Med 1994;331:10-5.

37. Greenberg R, Skornick Y, Kaplan O. Management of breast fibroadenomas. J Gen Intern Med 1998;3:640-5.

38. Sklair-Levy M, Sella T, Alweiss T, et al. Incidence and management of complex fibroadenomas. AJR Am J Roentgenol 2008;190:214-8.

39. Rosen PP. Fibroepithelial neoplasm. In: Rosen PP, editor. Rosen's breast pathology. 2nd ed. Philadelphia: Lippincott Williams & Wilkins; 2001. p.163-200.

40. Pinto J, Aguiar AT, Duarte H, et al. Simple and complex fibroadenomas are there any distinguishing sonographic features? J Ultrasound Med 2014;33:415-9.

41. Lozada JR, Burke KA, Maguire A, et al. Myxoid fibroadenomas differ from conventional fibroadenomas: a hypothesis-generating study. Histopathology 2017; 71:626-34.

42. Koerner FC. Myxoid fibroadenoma. In diagnostic problems in breast pathology. Philadelphia: W.B. Saunders; 2009. p. 321-7.

43. Koerner FC. Phyllodes tumor. In: Koerner FC, editor. Diagnostic Problems in Breast Pathology. Philadelphia, PA: Saunders, Elsevier; 2009. pp. 329-41.

44. Courcoutsakis NA, Tatsi C, Patronas NJ, et al. The complex of myxomas, spotty skin pigmentation and endocrine overactivity (carney complex): imaging findings with clinical and pathological correlation. Insights Imaging

2013;4:119-33.

45. Klinger K, Bhimani C, Shames J, et al. Fibroadenoma: from imaging evaluation to treatment. J Am Osteopath Coll Radiol 2019;8:17-30.

46. Edwards T, Jaffer S, Szabo JR, et al. Cellular Fibroadenoma on Core Needle Biopsy: Management recommendations for the radiologist. Clin Imaging 2016;40:587-90.

47. Lawton TJ, Acs G, Argani P, et al. Interobserver variability by pathologists in the distinction between cellular fibroadenomas and phyllodes tumors. Int J Surg Pathol 2014;22:695-8.

48. Foster ME, Garrahan N, Williams S. Fibroadenoma of the breast: a clinical and pathological study. J R Coll Surg Edinb 1988;33:16-9.

49. Sewell CW. Pathology of benign and malignant breast disorders. Radiol Clin North Am 1995;33:1067-84.

50. Lanyi M. Diagnosis and differential diagnosis of breast calcifications. New York, NY: Springer-Verlag; 1988. p. 145-56.

51. Morris EA. Breast magnetic resonance imaging lexicon. In: Morris EA, Liberman L, editors. Breast MRI. New York- NY: Springer; 2005. p. 51-78.

52. Dyer NH, Bridger JE, Taylor RS: Cystosarcoma phylloides. Br J Surg. 1966, 53:450-455. 10.1002/bjs.1800530517

53. Buchanan EB: Cystosarcoma phyllodes and its surgical management. Am Surgeon. 1995, 61:350-355.

54. Müller JP: Ueber den feinern Bau und die Formen der krankhaften Geschwülste . von Dr Johannes Müller..g. reimer. 1838.

55. Azzopardi JG, Chepick OF, Hartmann WH, et al: The World Health Organization histological typing of breast tumors-second edition. Am J Clin Pathol. 1982, 78:806-816.

56. Cheng SP, Chang YC, Liu TP, et al: Phyllodes tumor of the breast: the challenge persists. World J Surg. 2006, 30:1414-1421. 10.1007/s00268-005-

0786-2

57. Chaney AW, Pollack A, Mcneese MD, et al: Primary treatment of cystosarcoma phyllodes of the breast. Cancer. 2000, 89:1502-1511.

58. Barth RJ, Wells WA, Mitchell SE, et al: A prospective, multi-institutional study of adjuvant radiotherapy after resection of malignant phyllodes tumors. Ann Surg Oncol. 2009, 16:2288- 2294.

59. News on non-metastatic breast tumors; CNGOF 2013.

60. Belkacemi Y, Bousquet G, Marsiglia H, Ray-Coquard I, Magne N, Malard Y et al. Phyllodes tumor of the breast. Int J Radiat Oncol Biol Phys 2008;70:492-500.

61. Bernstein L, Deapen D, Ross RK: The descriptive epidemiology of malignant cystosarcoma phyllodes tumors of the breast. Cancer. 1993, 71:3020-3024.

62. Wang Y, Zhu J, Gou J, et al: Phyllodes tumors of the breast in 2 sisters: case report and review of literature. Medicine. 2017, 96:e8552.

63. Spitaleri G, Toesca A, Botteri E, et al: Breast phyllodes tumor: a review of literature and a single center retrospective series analysis. Crit Rev Oncol/Hematol. 2013, 88:427-436.

64. Pantoja E, Llobet RE, Lopez E: Gigantic cystosarcoma phyllodes in a man with gynecomastia Archives of Surgery. 1976, 111:611.

65. Cohn-Cedermark G, Rutqvist LE, Rosendahl I, Silfversward C: Prognostic factors incystosarcoma phyllodes. A clinicopathologic study of 77 patients. Cancer. 1991, 68:2017-2022.

66. Teo JY, Cheong CS, Wong CY: Low local recurrence rates in young Asian patients with phyllodes tumours: less is more. ANZ J Surg. 2012, 82:325-328.

67. Chua CL, Thomas A, Ng BK: Cystosarcoma phyllodes-Asian variations. Aust NZ J Surg. 1988, 58:301-305.

68. Jones AM, Mitter R, Springall R, et al: A comprehensive genetic profile of phyllodes tumours of the breast detects important mutations, intra-tumoral

genetic heterogeneity and new genetic changes on recurrence. J Pathol. 2008, 214:533-544.

69. Foucar CE, Hardy A, Siziopikou KP, et al: A mother and daughter with phyllodes tumors of the breast. Clin Breast Cancer. 2012, 12:373-377. 10.1016/j.clbc.2012.07.011

70. Wang Y, Zhu J, Gou J, et al: Phyllodes tumors of the breast in 2 sisters: case report and review of literature. Medicine. 2017, 96:e8552.

71. Matar N, Soumani A, Noun M, et al ; [Phyllodes tumors of the breast. Forty one cases.] J GynecolObstetBiolReprod1997 ;26 :32R6.78.

72. Linquist KD, Van Heerden JA. Recurrent and metastatic cystosarcoma phyllodes. Am JSur 1982; 144 :341.

73. Zurrida S, Bartoli C, Galimberti V, Squicciarini P, Delledonne V, Veronesi P, Bono A, de Palo G, Salvadori B. Which therapy for unexpected phyllode tumour of the breast? European Journal of Cancer 1992 ;28 :654-7.

74. Kapiris I, Nasiri N, A'Hern R, Healy V, Gui GP. Outcome and predictive factors of local recurrence and distant metastases following primary surgical treatment of high-grade malignant phyllodes tumours of the breast. European Journal of Surgical Oncology: the Journal of the European Society of Surgical Oncology and the British Association of Surgical Oncology 2001;27:723-30.

75. Mokbel K, Price RK, Mostafa CA, Wells CA, Carpenter R: Phyllodes tumour of the breast: a retrospective analysis of 30 cases. Breast. 1999, 8:278-281. 10.1054/brst.1999.0058

76. Jang JH, Choi MY, Lee SK, et al: Clinicopathologic risk factors for the local recurrence of phyllodes tumors of the breast. Ann Surg Oncol. 2012, 19:2612-2617.

77. Tan PH, Thike AA, Tan WJ, et al. Predicting clinical behaviour of breast phyllodes tumours: a nomogram based on histological criteria and surgical margins. J Clin Pathol. 2012; 65:69-76.

78. Parker SJ, Harries SA: Phyllodes tumours. Postgrad Med J. 2001, 77:428-435. 10.1136/pmj.77.909.428

79. Sheen-Chen SM, Chou FF, Chen WJ: Cystosarcoma phylloides of the breast: a review of clinical, pathological and therapeutic option in 18 cases. Int Surg. 1991, 76:101-104.

80. Pandey M, Mathew A, Kattoor J, et al: Malignant phyllodes tumor. Breast J. 2001, 7:411-416. 10.1046/j.1524-4741.2001.07606x.

81. Tardivon A et al. Imagerie de la femme : sénologie. Pathology-imaging correlations. 2014 ; 1-59.

82. Yanhong Zhang and Celina G. Kleer. Phyllodes Tumor of the Breast: Histopathologic Features, Differential Diagnosis, and Molecular/Genetic Updates. Archives of Pathology & Laboratory Medicine, vol. 140, no. 7, July 2016, pp. 665-671.

83. Reinfuss M, Mitus J, Duda K, et al: The treatment and prognosis of patients with phyllodes tumor of the breast: an analysis of 170 cases. Cancer. 1996, 77:910-916.

84. Lakhani SR: WHO Classification of Tumours of the Breast. International Agency for Research on Cancer, 2012.

85. Tan BY, Acs G, Apple SK, et al: Phyllodes tumours of the breast: a consensus review Histopathology. 2016, 68:5-21. 10.1111/his.12876.

86. Chen WH, Cheng SP, Tzen CY, et al: Surgical treatment of phyllodes tumors of the breast: retrospective review of 172 cases. J Surg Oncol. 2005, 91:185-194. 10.1002/jso.20334.

87. Liberman L, Bonaccio E, Hamele-Bena D, et al. Benign and malignant phyllodes tumors: mammographic and sonographic findings. Radiology 1996;198:121e4.

88. Chao TC, Lo YF, Chen SC, Chen MF. Phyllodes tumors of the breast. Eur Radiol.1 jan 2003 ; 13(1) :88-93

89. Cole-Beuglet C, Soriano R, Kurtz AB, et al. Ultrasound, x-ray mammography and histopathology of cystosarcoma phylloides. Radiology 1983;146:481e6.

90. Buchberger W,Strasser K, Heim K, Muller E Schrocksnadel H. Phylloides tumor: findings on mammography, sonography, and aspiration cytology in 10 cases. AJR Am J Roentgenol. Oct 1991; 157(4):715-9.

91. McNicholas MM, Mercer PM, Miller JC, McDermott EW, O'Higgins NJ, MacErlean DP. Color Doppler sonography in the evaluation of palpable breast masses. AJR Am J Roentgenol. 1993; 161: 765±771.

92. Wiratkapun C, Piyapan P, Lertsithichai P, Larbcharoensub N. Fibroadenoma versus phyllodes tumor:distinguishing factors in patients diagnosed with fibroepithelial lesions after a core needle biopsy. DiagnInterv Radiol. 2014; 20: 27±33.

93. Itoh A, Ueno E, Tohno E, Kamma H, Takahashi H, Shiina T, et al. Breast disease: clinical application of US elastography for diagnosis. Radiology 2006; 239: 341350.

94. Nunes LW, Schnall MD, Siegelman ES, et al: Diagnostic performance characteristics of architectural features revealed by high spatial-resolution MR imaging of the breast. Am J Roentgenol. 1997, 169:409-415. 10.2214/ajr.169.2.9242744

95. Rayzah M, Ryu JM, Lee JE, et al: Preoperative breast magnetic resonance imaging for the assessment of the size of ductal carcinoma in situ. J Breast Dis. 2016, 4:7784.

96. Tan H, Zhang S, Liu H, Peng W, Li R, Gu Y, Wang X, Mao J, Shen X. Imaging findings in phyllodes tumors of the breast. Eur J Radiol. 2012 Jan;81(1):e62-9.

97. Plaza MJ, Swintelski C, Yaziji H, Torres-Salichs M, Esserman LE. Phyllodes tumor: review of key imaging characteristics. Breast Dis. 2015;35(2):79-86.

98. Yabuuchi H, Soeda H, Matsuo Y, Okafuji T, Eguchi T, Sakai S, Kuroki S, Tokunaga E, Ohno S, Nishiyama K, Hatakenaka M, Honda H. Phyllodes tumor

of the breast: correlation between MR findings and histologic grade. Radiology. 2006 Dec;241(3):702-9.

99. Farria DM, Gorczyea DP, Barsky SH, Sinha S, Basset LW. Benign phyllodes tumor of the breast; MR imaging features. AJR. 1996;167:187-189.

1 00.Ogawa Y, Nishioka A, Tsuboi N, Yoshida D, Inomata T, Yoshida S, Moriki T, Toki T. Dynamic MR appearance of benign phyllodes tumor of the breast in a 20- year-old woman. Radiat Med. 1997 Jul-Aug;15(4):247-50.

101. Tse GM, Cheung HS, Pang LM, Chu WC, Law BK, Kung FY, Yeung DK. Characterization of lesions of the breast with proton MR spectroscopy: comparison of carcinomas, benign lesions, and phyllodes tumors. AJR Am J Roentgenol. 2003 Nov;181(5):1267-72.

102. Durand JC.E'coulements mamelonnaires. Encycl Med Chir (Éditions Scientifiques et Médicales Elsevier, Paris), Gynécologie, 812-A-20, 1997 : 1-4.

103. Woods ER, Helvie MA, Ikeda DM, Mandell SH, Chapel KL, Adler DD et al. Solitary breast papilloma: comparison of mammographic, galactographic and pathologic findings. Am J Roentgenol 1992; 159 (3): 487-49.

104. Collins LC, Schnitt SJ. Papillary lesions of the breast: selected diagnostic and management issues. Histopathology. 2008 Jan;52(1):20-9.

105. Kussaibi H, De Roquancourt A, Bertheau P. Atlas des l√Osions mammaires. www.anapath.org. 2010.

106. Courtillot C. Benign breast diseases. J Mammary Gland Biol Neoplasia 2005;10:325-35. Heywang-Krunnner SH, Schreer I, Dershaw DD. Benign tumors. Diagnostic breast imaging. 1st ed. Stuttgart: Thieme; 1997. P 180-6.

107. Woods ER. Solitary breast papilloma: comparison of mammographic, galactographic, and pathologic findings. AJR Am J Roentgenol. 1992;159:487-91.

108. Eiada R, Chong J, Kulkarni S, Goldberg F, Muradali D. Papillary lesions of the breast: MRI, ultrasound, and mammographic appearances. AJR Am J Roentgenol. 2012 Feb;198(2):264-71.

109. Jagmohan P, Pool FJ, Putti TC, Wong J. Papillary lesions of the breast: imaging findings and diagnostic challenges. Diagn Interv Radiol. 2013 Nov-Dec;19(6):471-8 .

110. Kihara M, Miyauchi A. Intracystic papilloma of the breast forming a giant cyst. Breast Cancer. 2010;17:68-70.

111. Duan G, Xu YK, Deng HJ, Huang CT. Mammography and magnetic resonance imaging for diagnosis of the intraductal papilloma of the breast. Nan Fang Yi Ke Da Xue Xue Bao. 2009;29:1643-6.

112. Amin AL, Purdy AC, Mattingly JD, Kong AL, Termuhlen PM. Benign breast disease. Surg Clin North Am. 2013 Apr;93(2):299-308.

113. Manfrin E. Benign breast lesions at risk of developing cancer-a challenging problem in breast cancer screening programs: five years' experience of the Breast Cancer Screening Program in Verona (1999- 2004). Cancer. 2009;115:499-507.

114. Jaffer S, Nagi C, Bleiweiss IJ. Excision is indicated for intraductal papilloma of the breast diagnosed on core needle biopsy. Cancer. 2009;115:2837-43.

115. Ko ES. Sonographic changes after removing all benign breast masses with sonographically guided vacuum-assisted biopsy. Acta Radiol. 2009;50:968-74.

116. Zhang S, Huo L, Arribas E, Middleton LP. Adenomyoepithelioma of the breast with associated atypical lobular hyperplasia: a previously unrecognized association with management implications. Ann Diagn Pathol. 2015 Feb;19(1):20-3.

117. Zafrani B, Aubriot M H, Mouret E.et al High sensitivity and specificity of

immunohistochemistry for the detection of hormone receptors in breast carcinoma: comparison with biochemical determination in a prospective study of 793 cases. Histopathology. 2000;37536-545.

118. Howlett DC, Mason CH, Biswas S, et al. Adenomyoepithelioma of the breast: spectrum of disease with associated imaging and pathology. AJR Am J Roentgenol. 2003;180:799.

119. Lee JH, Kim SH, Kang BJ, et al. Ultrasonographic features of benign adenomyoepithelioma of the breast. Korean J Radiol 2010;11:522.

120. Tukel S, Ustuner E, Aytac SK. Adenomyoepithelioma of the breast. J Ultrasound Med. 2001;20: 1021.

121. Ruiz-Delgado ML, Lopez-Ruiz JA, Eizaguirre B, et al. Benign adenomyoepithelioma of the breast: imaging findings mimicking malignancy and histopathological features. Acta Radiol. 2007;48:27.

122. Adejolu M, Wu Y, Santiago L, et al. Adenomyoepithelial tumors of the breast: imaging findings with histopathologic correlation. AJR Am J Roentgenol. 2011;197:184.

1 23.Stavros AT. Ultrasound of solid breast nodules: distinguishing benign from malignant. In: Stavros AT, editor. Breast Ultrasound. Philadelphia: Lippincott Williams & Wilkins. 2004, p 445.

1 24.Vuitch MF, Rosen PP, Erlandson RA. Pseudoangiomatous hyperplasia of mammary stroma. Hum Pathol 1986;17:185-91.

1 25.Sng KK, Tan SM, Mancer JFK, Tay KH. The contrasting presentation and management of pseudoangiomatous stromal hyperplasia of the breast. Singapore Med J 2008;49:82-5.

126. Ferreira M, Albarracin CT, Resetkova E. Pseudoangiomatous stromal hyperplasia tumor: a clinical, radiologic and pathologic study of 26 cases. Mod Pathol 2008;21:201-7.

127. Mansouri D, Mrad K, Sassi S, Driss-Fourati M, Abbes I, Koobaa-Mahjoub W, et al. Pseudoangiomatous hyperplasia of the mammary stroma. Ann Pathol 2004;24:179-82.

128.Okashi K, Ogawa H, Suwa H, Saiga T, Kobayashi H. A case of nodular Pseudoangiomatous stromal hyperplasia (PASH). Breast Cancer 2006;13:349-53.

129 Powell CM, Cranor ML, Rosen PP. Pseudoangiomatous stromal hyperplasia (PASH). A mammary stromal tumor with myofibroblastic differentiation. Am J Surg Pathol 1995;19: 270-7.

130.Ibrahim RE, Sciotto CG, Weidner N. Pseudoangiomatous hyperplasia of mammary stroma. Some observations regarding its clinicopathologic spectrum. Cancer 1989;63:1154-60.

131. Lee JS, Oh HS, Min KW. Mammary pseudoangiomatous stromal hyperplasia presenting as an axillary mass. Breast 2005;14:61-4.

132. Taira N, Ohsumi S, Aogi K, Maeba T, Kawamura S, Nishimura R, et al. Nodular pseudoangiomatous stromal hyperplasia of mammary stroma in a case showing rapid tumor growth. Breast Cancer 2005;12:331-6.

133. Cohen MA, Morris EA, Rosen PP, Dershaw DD, Liberman L, Abramson AF. Pseudoangiomatous stromal hyperplasia: Mammographic, sonographic, and clinical patterns. Breast Imaging 1996;198: 117-20.

134. Celliers L, Wong DD, Bourke A. Pseudoangiomatous stromal hyperplasia: a study of the mammographic and sonographic features. Clin Radiol. 2010 Feb;65(2):145-9 .

135. Charpin C, Mathoulin MP, Andrac L, et al. Reappraisal of breast hamartomas. A morphological study of 41 cases. Pathol Res Pract 1994;190:362-371

136. Arrigoni MG, Dockerty MB, Judd ES. The identification and treatment of mammary hamartoma. Surg Gynecol Obstet 1971

1 37.Oueslati, S, Salem A, Chebbi A, Mhiri S, Kribi L, Ben Romdhane K, et al. Hamartoma of the breast. Imagerie de la Femme. 2007; 17(1):19-25.

138. Hogeman K-E, Ostberg G. Three cases of postlactational breast tumour of a peculiar type. Acta Pathol Microbiol Scand 1968;73:169-176.

139. Linell F, Ostberg G, Soderstrom J, et al. Breast hamartomas. An important entity

in mammary pathology. Virchows Arch [A] 1979;383:253-264.

140. Boyer B, Graef C. Hamartoma of the breast: a rare b√Onigne tumor of mammographic diagnosis. La Presse M√Odicale. 2007 ; 36 (12):1999-2000.

141. Kaplan L, Walts AE. Benign chondrolipomatous tumor of the human female breast. Arch Pathol Lab Med 1977;101:149-151.

142. Hayashi H, Ito T, Matsushita K, et al. Mammary hamartoma: immunohistochemical study of two adenolipomas and one variant with cartilage, smooth muscle and myoepithelial proliferation. Pathol Int 1996;46:60-65.

143. Daya D, Trus T, D'Souza TJ, et al. Hamartoma of the breast an underrecognized breast lesion. A clinicopathologic and radiographic study of 25 cases. Am J Clin Pathol 1995;103:685-689.

144. Fisher C, Hanby AM, Robinson L, et al. Mammary hamartoma - a review of 35 cases. Histopathology 1992;20:99-106.

145. Wahner-Roedler DL, Sebo TJ, Gisvold JJ. Hamartomas of the breast: clinical, radiologic, and pathologic manifestations. Breast J 2001;7:101-105.

146. Coyne J, Hobbs FM, Boggis C, et al. Lobular carcinoma in a mammary hamartoma. J Clin Pathol 1992;45:936-937.

147. Mester J, Simmons RM, Vazquez MF, et al. In situ and infiltrating ductal carcinoma arising in a breast hamartoma. AJR Am J Roentgenol 2000;175:64-

66.

148. Anani PA, Hessler C. Breast hamartoma with invasive ductal carcinoma. Report of two cases and review of the literature. Pathol Res Pract 1996;192:1187-1194.

149. Tse GMK, Law BKB, Ma TKF, et al. Ductal carcinoma in situ arising in mammary hamartoma. J Clin Pathol 2002;55: 541-542.

150. Lee EH, Wylie EJ, Bourke AG, De Boer WB. Invasive ductal carcinoma arising in a breast hamartoma: two case reports and a review of the literature. Clin Radiol. 2003;58(1):80-83.

151. Conant EF, Brennecke CM. Mosby Inc; 2006. Breast imaging, case review.

152. Chao TC, Chao HH, Chen MF. Sonographic features of breast hamartomas. J Ultrasound Med. 2007;26:447-452.

153. Presazzi A, Di Giulio G, Calliada F. Breast hamartoma: ultrasound, elastosonographic, and mammographic features. Mini pictorial essay. J Ultrasound. 2015;18:373-377.

154. Sanal HT, Ersoz N, Altinel O, Unal E, Can C. Giant hamartoma of the breast. Breast J. 2006;12:84-85.

155. Rohini A, Prachi K, Bhargavi V. Multimodality imaging of giant breast hamartoma with pathological correlation. Int J Basic Appl Med Sci. 2014;4:278-281.

156. Park SY, Oh KK, Kim EK, Son EJ, Chung WH. Sonographic findings of breast hamartoma: emphasis on compressibility. Yonsei Med J. 2003;44:847-854.

157. Wong KW, Ho WC, Wong TT. MRI of muscular hamartoma of the breast. Australas Radiol. 2002;46:441-443.

158. Posadilla MA,Torres LP, Plaza FJ, Castañón RR, de Francisco TG, Olcoz Goñi JL. Importance of magnetic resonance imaging in the diagnosis of multiple small biliary hamartomas. Gastroenterol Hepatol. 2006 Jun-

Jul;29(6):378-9.

159. Nam SY, Han BK, Lee S, Lee K. MR findings of hamartoma of the breast: a report of two cases. J Korean Soc Magn Resonance Med. 2012;16(3):271-275.

160. Boufettal, H., Mahdaoui, S., Noun, M., Hermas, S., & Samouh, N. Breast hamartoma. Feuillets de Radiologie. 2010 ; 50(4), 189-191.

161. Brenner RJ, Karlan MS. Recurrent amyloid mass of the breast: mammographic and ultrasonographic features. J Le Sein 1995; 5 (1): 29-31.

162. Hecht AH, Tan A, Shen JF. Case report: primary systemic amyloidosis presenting as breast masses, mammographically simulating carcinoma. Clin Radiol 1991; 4: 123-124.

1 63.Sabate J.M., Clotet M., Torrubia S.: Radiologic evaluation of breast disorders related to pregnancy and lactation. Radiographics. 2007; 27 (Suppl. 1): pp. S101- S124.

164.   Cholot M, Dang-Tran KD, Castelain CS. Postpartum inflammatory breast tumor: necrotic lactating adenoma. Imagerie de la femme 2007;17:40-5.

165. Baker TP, Lenert JT, Parker J. Lactating adenoma: a diagnosis of exclusion. Breast J 2001;5:354-7.

166. Rosen PP, Holmes G, Lesser ML, Kinne DW, Bealtie J. Juvenile papillomatosis and breast carcinoma. Cancer 1985; 55: 1345-1352.

167. Kersschot EA, Hermans M, Pauwells C, Gildemyn G, Chabeau P, De Vos L et al. Juvenile papillomatosis of the breast. Sonographic appearance. Radiology 1988 ; 169 : 631-633.

168. Bazzocchi F, Santini D, Martinelli G, Piccaluga A, Taffurelli M, Grassiagli A et al. Juvenile papillomatosis (epitheliosis) of the breast. A clinical and pathological study of 13 cases. Am J Clin Pathol 1986 ; 86 (6) : 745-748.

169. Le Treut A, Testard S, Trojani M, De Mascarel I, Dilhuydy MH. Juvenile papillomatosis: about four observations. J Le Sein 1991; 1 (1): 17-21.

170. Fontanges M, Barreau B, Dilhuydy MH, De Mascarel I. Sonographic aspects of juvenile papillomatosis. JEMU 1994; 15 (16): 348-351.

171.Santos-Magadán S, López-Casañas AM, Martínez-González J, Taborda Ramírez LF, Moreno-Torres A, Carreira-Gómez C. Juvenile papillomatosis of the breast. Clinical Cases. 2017. Eurorad.

172.Barreau B, Dilhuydy MH, Fontanges M. Juvenile papillomatosis of the breast: US aspect - An approach to diagnosis. In :MadjarH,TeubnerJ, HackeloerBeds. Breast Ultrasound Update. Basel : Kager, 1994 : 208-213.

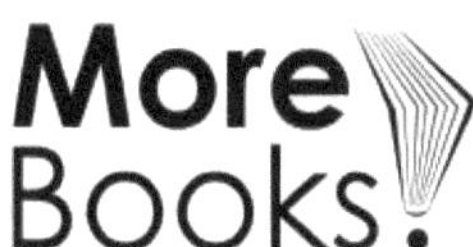

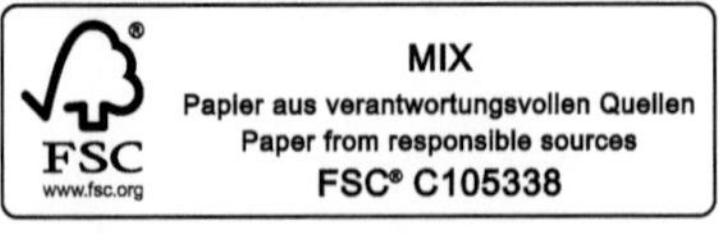

Printed by Books on Demand GmbH, Norderstedt / Germany